"Finally, a practical guidebook to help understand and improve kid's eating habits."

—**Lee Constantine**, Cofounder/CMO at Publishizer

"*Food Fight* is a must-have for any family looking for healthy and fun ways to feed their kids, picky eaters or not. Chef Gigi's culinary genius and her ability to understand and feed people of any age are beautifully blended in this book. The strategies presented are right on the money and I love the long list of easy, fun, healthy and super child friendly recipes. Already a staple in my kitchen library!"

—**Vanessa Silva**, Founder / Culinary Artistas,
Creative Cooking Classes for Kids
San Francisco, Ca.

"*Food Fight* focuses on the most difficult time of day for many parents: mealtime. Learn how to cope with picky eaters and serve your youngsters nutritious meals they will actually eat. You'll even discover some fun, activities you can do with your children! Chef Gigi offers great ideas to promote healthful eating and improve parent-child relationships."

—**Diane Flynn Keith**, Homeschool Specialist and
Author of *Car Schooling*, San Francisco Bay Area

"Delicious! We savored the recipes, strategies and information fed to us as if we were guests in Chef Gigi's own kitchen. Chef Gigi breaks down tantrums with taste and puts style on strategy. Make lunch, not war will be the new rallying cry for our toddler's mealtime. *Food Fight* guarantees a win for everyone seated at the table. Brava, Chef Gigi. "

—Chef Tony Spatafora, Host of "Dish It Out!"

"Gigi is wonderfully passionate about healthy food! She's upbeat, hard working and always looking for a fresh angle when it comes to culinary challenges like getting little ones to eat their vegetables. With her help, we have a toddler who eats vegetables and looks forward to helping prepare dinner. Her guidance has been invaluable as a first-time mom and this book makes it available to me at any hour, every day. "

—Heather Vega, Director Larson Communications and Jamison's Mom

"As a personal chef who has cooked for lots of people with picky children, I've seen how stressful it can be for both parents and kids. In *Food Fight*, Chef Gigi provides true solutions to a frustrating dilemma. She covers it all, from the psychology of what makes a child a picky eater to kids nutrition-she touches on food intolerances, and adds real-life strategies, including delicious recipes! *Food Fight* is an absolute must have for anyone who struggles with family mealtimes."

—Simone Miller, Author of *The Zenbelly Cookbook, Paleo Soups & Stews*, and Coauthor of *The New Yiddish Kitchen*

"Chef Gigi is a voice of reassurance and reason, as she encourages parents to set down tired negotiation tropes (get ready to say goodbye to the one-bite rule!) and sets us up for meal-time success with strategies for developing positive eating habits right from the get-go."

—Lindsay-Jean Hard, Josephine's mother and Author of *Cooking with Scraps*

"*Food Fight* is chock full of practical and helpful solutions for parents who struggle with mealtimes."

—Chef Miriam Russell-Wadleigh, General Manager, Guckenheimer, Samsung's First Cafe

"With her culinary background, Chef Gigi teaches you how to make quick and easy dishes that use professional techniques. Using taste science, she shows you how to make your kid-friendly dishes match the taste profiles that young palates are looking for. "

—Michael Kalanty, Award-winning Author, *How To Bake Bread: The Five Families of Bread*®

"This book is perfect for my daughter. She has improved dramatically not only in her eating habits but also in her overall health. She is much more outgoing with regards to trying new foods, and I am much more motivated to cooperate at mealtimes too, Chef Gigi. Thank you!"

—Olive's parent, San Francisco, California

"Both of my children love working with me on the family meal now. My son has made wonderful improvements, not only in active listening; I've made some changes myself with my level of confidence in parenting. My daughter has moved up to enjoying our new foods day of the week, and has discovered a few things she has added to her food repertoire. Thank you so much—our mealtimes are much easier after applying some of Chef Gigi's techniques!"

—Jackson's grandmother, Los Angeles, California

"We had the 'one-bite rule' at our home and realized it is a control issue after working with Chef Gigi. We actually have used a few of her tips and it really does make a difference. Not to mention Gigi taught us how to use closed-ended choices—now, our lives are a bit easier. Thank you for putting us in check, Gigi; we were tired of being short-order cooks!"

—Joseph, father of three, Hillsborough, California

Food Fight:
For Parents of Picky Eaters
by Chef Gigi Gaggero

© Copyright 2018 Chef Gigi Gaggero

ISBN 978-1-63393-662-1

Published by

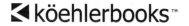 köehlerbooks™

210 60th Street
Virginia Beach, VA 23451
800–435–4811
www.koehlerbooks.com

FOOD FIGHT

FOR PARENTS OF PICKY EATERS

CHEF GIGI GAGGERO

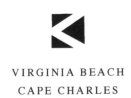

VIRGINIA BEACH
CAPE CHARLES

For Gabrielle and Dakota.

*My teachers, I never understood
what true love was until I met you!*

TABLE OF CONTENTS

AUTHOR'S NOTE

Here I am, mid-life, and not for one moment did I think I would add "published book author" to my résumé. My successful culinary career has been challenging yet satisfying. I've heard, "The road to success never comes with ease." I am confirming that.

For my entire life and career, I have been in constant motion—climbing the metaphorical summit, repeatedly losing my footing, yet gliding up and down the mountain steadily. Some years felt as though for every two steps up, I slipped back three. Reaching the top, I would dust myself off, stand tall, breathe deeply, and boldly survey the land, only to find myself at the base of yet another mountain.

As I matured in my career and as a woman, I realized that my greatest triumphs came from my failures. I finally understand that I had to master my inaccuracies in order to grow.

Today, I am a little wiser, a little stronger, and much more of age. I believe my fruitful career might not have happened without those who supported me along the arduous expedition. Although alone in my daily journey, my trek has been fortified by a succession of others.

This book is for those who fed me, drank with me, cried with me, hugged and believed in me. Those who stood by my side and knew I could reach the summit before I knew I could. Those who have been with me for three months or thirty years! You strengthened me to continue in one way or another. This book is a representation of your support, for which I am eternally grateful.

Thank you:

Gretchen Aberg

Liz and Aaron Anchando

Chef Gwen C. Beltran and family

Chef Brett Byram Beza

Dan Boardman Jr.

An and Patti Chen and family

Doris Cook

Lee Constantine

Lori Nicole DeAvilla

Lisa De Zordo

Rose Domingo

Richard Donati

Chef Elianna Friedmanm

Florence Gaggero

Al Gerona

Laura Hansen

Eric, Suyun, Adam, Collin and Ethan Kim

Alice and Bill Leary

Chef Francisco Javier Martinez

Maria Milik and family

Chef Simone Miller

Ross Meyer

Ed and Irma Medina

Adela Padron

Josephine Park

Chef Pesha Perlsweig

Terry Post

Marc and Wenonalani Randolph

Elisa All Schmitz

Anne Stone

Chef Suji Kong

John Koehler

David "Bro" Topacio

Chef Cristina Topham

Rhoda Toshimitsu

Chef Heidi Rae Weinstein

INTRODUCTION

Congratulations on taking this first step toward food fight freedom. If you're reading this, you must be at a point where mealtimes are being held hostage and everyone in your home tries to avoid the dreaded dinnertime nightmare. As children become more aware of the world around them, they become discerning eaters. Generally, I hear parents say, "When my child was a baby, she would eat anything!" As a seasoned parent, I know agreeability usually doesn't last. By age two, children have a routine of familiar, safe foods, and once they have established a familiar routine, they hesitate to try anything new or different.

A big challenge I hear about all the time is introducing new foods to older kids. Children from seven to ten years old have already established likes and dislikes and how they will consume foods. Even if we know they will enjoy a certain food, this age group usually requires additional steps before they will actually taste and accept the food into their repertoire. I've tested several fun techniques over the years that will help you engender a curiosity about new foods with this age group. Hopefully these techniques will help you entice interest and the child will step forward and explore a new menu item.

To get the most out of this book, I will suggest positive parenting techniques such as closed-ended choices and journaling. Educate yourself on what foods and introductions are not working with your child. Write them down. And last but not least, prepare for battle by briefly understanding the science of flavor. Identify your child's preferred tastes. And, while managing all of this, don't forget to give yourself a break. Parenting is not an easy post, and dealing with a picky eater certainly adds to your already overbooked task capacity.

My hope is to support you in abandoning a few of the very common yet ultimately unsuccessful tactics that parents use to get their toddlers to eat.

You will also learn how much your child actually needs to eat to stay healthy (which will reassure most of you). I also provide how-to tips for creating routine and structure.

Please read all the material and let the information digest. Do not try to implement a plan until you get through the whole book. By then, you will have all the knowledge you need to start making positive changes for you, your child, and the rest of the family. Soon everyone will begin enjoying some much deserved stress-free family mealtimes.

The knowledge presented in this book is not intended to diagnose, treat, cure, or prevent any disease or food intolerances. All information is intended for your general awareness only and is not a substitute for medical advice or treatment of specific medical conditions. Discuss your child's eating patterns with a healthcare provider or your child's pediatrician before you determine what is right for your family.

Chapter One

WHY ARE SOME CHILDREN PICKY EATERS?

Like all of us, children want to feel that they have some control and power over their lives. Often they do the reverse of what is asked of them just to exercise power. One way a child exerts his power and control is through food. This usually works. It's unreasonable to force a child to eat. We all know children who refuse to eat their vegetables or whatever it is they claim to dislike. They're willing to sit at the table for an additional thirty minutes or more while the parents wait for them to eat. Realistically, if you pay attention, you can see it has more to do with power and control than being a picky eater. The old oppositional behavior trick will usually be your first clue, comparable to potty training or bedtime troubles. Peer pressure can be another factor. Children will follow the displays of their peers. If you have more than one child at the table, you will need to up your food fight strategy and stick to it.

Our sense of taste tells our brains which of the four basic

tastes we are experiencing: sweet, salty, sour or bitter. If a child develops a preference for one of those flavors from an early age, odds are she will stick to foods with similar flavor profiles. People have a genetic preference for sweet and salty and a genetic displeasure for bitter and sour. Children list sweet foods like ice cream as their favorites and, as you could probably guess, bitter foods like brussels sprouts and spinach as their least favorites. Dr. James Keaney, a practicing physician in the San Francisco Bay area, confirms that children, like adults, have a natural aversion to bitter foods, which may be a survival measure. Most naturally-occurring poisons taste bitter and initiate a gag reflex. Therefore, the child is not to blame; it's our body's natural defense. Some flavors and even textures may take longer to be accepted than others. Over time, food fights will disappear if the parent remembers to utilize a few proven techniques, flavor enhancers, and a big dash of fortitude.

Often we blur taste with smell. Very little of what we taste is actually experienced on our taste buds. The experience of flavor is a combination of smell, sight, touch and texture. Keep in mind that all those senses contribute to children accepting food. Because flavor is a combination of smell and taste, with smell often being the more important factor, most kids will choose foods by smell first.

Spaghetti is a favorite choice for picky eaters because it contains both salty and sweet elements. Spaghetti is garnished with alluring smell and, let's face it, spaghetti is fun to eat. The salty and sweet flavor combination is something the food world calls the "fifth sense" of taste on our tongues, the "umami" sense (/oo-mommy/). As a parent of a picky eater, umami might be your best ally. (See Chapter Nine: The Advanced Battle for more information on umami flavors.)

"Understanding umami mechanisms isn't just interesting, it's useful," says Edmund Rolls, DSc, a professor at the Oxford Centre for Computational Neuroscience who researches taste mechanisms and the brain. Understanding the science behind flavor is another tool to add to your arsenal. For instance, some children will not accept the flavor of nutrient-dense green vegetables. However, when enhanced with flavors of umami, the landscape of flavor changes, and for the better. Using the science behind flavor layered with techniques found in this book will certainly enhance your toolbox. One of the most important things to remember when engaging in a food fight pattern is to make sure the food tastes good.

Not all picky eaters are equal. Some kids will eat what others will not. Keep an open mind. If you scowl or comment negatively about food, the kids might too. I've added an array of interesting recipes at the end of this book that might run the gamut for all levels of eaters. Perhaps a few of them will add to your family's culinary repertoire.

Some children that are picky or selective eaters could be reacting to their own bodies' defense mechanisms. Children who are not speaking yet or have been identified as disabled or on the autistic spectrum might not be eating due to internal reactions to the foods. Your child's body will naturally reject certain foods for a multitude of reasons. This is a good time to begin identifying food allergies. If children react to certain foods, pay close attention. The body may be speaking or screaming for help. Observe these cues and keep a food journal. Maybe your child is pressing his belly against the dinner table. This might signal a bellyache.

Whatever foods are causing these reactions should stay off the menu forever. Look for symptoms such as nausea, stomach pain, low intestinal integrity, shortness of breath, or hives, just to name a few. This is unlike being a picky eater and should be identified as "food intolerance." If the digestive system alone rejects the food, finding it difficult to digest properly, seek help sooner than later. Along with other irritant reactions, sometimes intolerances are hard to immediately recognize. Observe, take notes, list the nuisance foods and the responses you see your child having, and get to a medical professional as soon as possible.

Have I created a picky eater?

All children are different. Some happily eat everything placed in front of them, and some have a repertoire of a half dozen foods they will eat. If you have more than one child, you might find that one is very picky and another eats almost anything. I'd like to say this is not the result of your parenting; however, the problem could be the way that many parents present or represent food. Very young children do better with finger foods and a variety of textures and colors served in small portions on their plates. A child's body does crave the nutrition it needs; refrain from presenting foods in a negative way or using bribing tools.

As parents, we learn that there are developmental reasons for everything related to our child's growth. Keep in mind that it is normal for kids between one and three years of age to poke at their food. Also, after a year of rapid growth, toddlers gain weight much slower and therefore require less food intake. The fact is, toddlers are always on the go and won't sit still for anything, including food. This will affect their eating patterns. Don't punish; teach.

If the child is forced to sit down at a table and be still during a meal, you will lose the battle. Each age range has different developmental characteristics and, unfortunately, at this age, sitting still is not one of them. Toddlers inherently snack their way through the day. This is more compatible with the busy explorer lifestyle than sitting down to a full-fledged feast. You should make smaller offerings throughout the day and more frequently. When this age group moves to older developmental styles and behaviors, you can start to introduce by bringing them to the family table and keeping them there. And remember that every child is different. Some children that are larger in stature will be working longer on their motor coordination. Don't compare.

As a parent, learning more about developmental stages and ages can really help you relax. Your job is simply to buy the right food, prepare it nutritiously (steamed rather than boiled, baked rather than fried) and serve it, creative or not. Trust yourself and leave the rest up to the youngsters. How much they eat, when they eat, and if they eat is mostly their responsibility. As a parent, part of emotional maturity is learning to take neither the credit nor the blame. This is a difficult level to achieve since, as parents, we are also about power and control. Food fight successes comes from designing and working within a closed-ended boundary model of household management.

Will my child starve if I don't insist he eats?

To my knowledge, no child has starved to death from his picky eating habits. It's easy for parents to feel apprehensive when their growing child isn't consuming the calories they feel his growing body requires. In most cases, if the child's height and weight are within the normal range, there is nothing to worry about. If you are worried, get reassurance from a physician. Children's bodies are small. They need smaller portion sizes and will eat up to six times a day. In fact, experts suggest an adult body should be fueled periodically throughout the day by six small meals containing 200 to 250 calories per meal. Eat with your child; don't just stand or sit there.

If you can, imagine your child's little body and visualize that the capacities are much less, and you will understand this concept better. Don't forget, most toddlers like to binge on one food at a time. They may eat only fruits one day and then only vegetables the next. Since erratic eating habits are as normal as a toddler mood swing, expect your child to eat well one day and practically nothing the next. Your child won't starve; they will eat when they are hungry. Aim for a nutritionally-balanced week, not a balanced day. All this is not to say that you shouldn't encourage toddlers and small children to eat well and develop healthy food habits. Based on my hands-on experience with children, I've developed several tactics to tempt little taste buds and minimize mealtime hassles.

According to the American Heart Association, the suggested caloric intakes are:

Toddlers from ages one to three years who are moderately active need between 900 and 1,400 calories a day.

Kids from four to eight years require an estimated 1,400 to 1,600 calories a day.

Kids from nine to thirteen years can vary based on gender. Moderately-active females should consume a minimum of 1,600 calories and males a minimum of 1,800 calories per day, unless they are very active sports enthusiasts.

Female athletes from nine to thirteen years old should consume a minimum of 1,800 calories per day and males should consume a minimum of 2,000.

Don't overfeed infants and young children. They usually self-regulate the calories they need each day. Children shouldn't be forced to finish meals if they aren't hungry, as they often vary caloric intake from meal to meal. Always introduce healthy foods and continue to offer them if they're initially refused. Omit introducing foods without healthy nutritional value simply to provide calories.

Serve a variety of fruits and vegetables daily, while limiting juice intake. Each meal should contain at least one fruit or vegetable. A female child's recommended fruit intake ranges from one cup per day between ages one and three to two cups for ages fourteen to eighteen. For a male, recommended vegetable intake ranges from two thirds of a cup a day at one year old to three cups for a fourteen-year-old.

As children grow, keep total fat intake between 30 and 35 percent of calories for children three years of age, and between 25 and 35 percent for children and adolescents four to fourteen years of age, with most fats coming from sources of polyunsaturated and monounsaturated fatty acids such as fish, nuts, and healthy vegetable oils.

Serve whole grain, high-fiber breads and cereals rather than refined grain products. Look for "whole grain" as the first ingredient on the food label and make at least half of your grain servings whole grain.

Introduce and regularly serve fish as an entrée. Avoid commercially-fried or baked fish that comes in a box ready to reheat. Avoid feeding your child empty calories at all costs. I know this sounds like a huge challenge, but I can tutor you, via my recipes, in how to cook an item like commercially bought fish sticks or fast food chicken nuggets in your own home in under thirty minutes. You will feel much better about feeding your family clean and free from artificial shelf stabilizers found in convenience foods. Cooking at home also gives your family the occasion to get involved in the process of preparing a family meal. Children are more likely to eat what they prepare.

Will my child always be a picky eater?

Most children grow out of their picking eating stage and grow up to be adults who consume a variety of foods. Some children will go through their whole childhood being difficult eaters. With others, it may only last a few months or a few years. Usually if we learn to relax and not make it a big issue, they will start to welcome new foods into their diet. With a few of the suggested methods in this book, you will have fun pioneering new foods for your child's repertoire. Some of these practices are so much fun that your children will grow up with fond memories of mealtimes and possibly pass them down to future generations.

Chapter Two

FOOD FIGHT STRATEGIES FOR CHILDREN

Ages One to Seven

We've all done it—pleaded with our toddler to try just one bite of a sandwich or conveyed that if he tries the soup he can have a treat or go on an outing. We are all guilty of letting him have a third glass of milk or juice between meals because at least then we are certain that something is in his little belly. We all think, *When he gets a bit older, he will eat.* The truth is, we are beat by the stubborn refusals and we just give in. "My kid's picky," we say while giving her last night's cheese pizza for breakfast, or "She only eats white food," while handing our preschooler a piece of French bread and butter with fruit for mealtime.

With all the bribing, manipulating, and even threatening consequences from no dessert to time-outs, we are still left feeling powerless against our pint-size, food-refusing child's strong will. Welcome to the seemingly never-ending food fight.

Toddler years are notorious for trying the patience of even the most calm and loving parents. Toddlers are trying to figure out who they are and how they fit in the world. No matter how much you control what your toddler cannot do, it is virtually impossible to force him to do things he has decided not to do. Eating is one of the few things that toddlers and preschoolers have some control over because we can't force them to chew and swallow. Like most power struggles, the more we worry, play games, threaten and bribe, the worse the encounter will become.

In order to shift this pattern, you must alter your feeding habits and set a new agenda of healthy food consumption for your children. In order to design a new, successful plan of action, first we should examine why the collective methods most parents use often don't work.

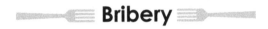

Bribery

What it looks like

"Eat the carrot, and Mommy will give you a cookie."

Bribing is, simply put, offering a reward for good behavior. In the food fight framework, many parents use a more desirable food as a bribe to get a child to eat a less desirable food.

Why we do it

Because it works sometimes—or, at least, it works to some degree. This approach can bring some measure of relief to parents who are terrified that their child isn't getting enough protein, carbohydrates or vegetables. Many children will force down a few bites of spaghetti in order to get the jelly donut that has been promised for dessert.

Parents, reality check. This technique is a quick fix, and it possibly becomes very labor intensive for you later as your picky eater grows.

Parent smart, not hard. In the long run, your actions and bribery choices will not teach your child about healthy eating habits. Instead of just sitting down and having a pleasurable meal, you will have to watch every bite or hold up the reward food to remind your toddler. It can be disruptive and can pull your attention away from your other children at the dinner table. If all your time and energy is dedicated to your fussy eater, it's time to declare a food fight!

Why it doesn't work

The leading setback with bribery is how it creates lists of negative and positive foods in the child's mind. Sweets and salty snacks, such as chips or candy, fall on the positive side, and almost everything else on the negative side. The same disadvantage occurs when we tell our children that they must finish their vegetables or other healthier versions of food before they acquire dessert. Ideally, the child should look at all foods as equal. Our child will still have likes and dislikes, and of course many of his "likes" will probably be sweets. By taking the "reward" out of those foods, the foods become less attractive, opening the way for additional healthful foods to become desirable. Why shouldn't sweet, creamy Greek yogurt topped with a sprinkling of cinnamon be something for the child to celebrate as enthusiastically as a dessert?

Threatening

What it looks like

"Eat your dinner, or you'll get a time out."

Threatening is essentially the same as bribing, just reversed. Instead of offering a reward for eating, we offer a punishment if they don't eat. Think about that. You are at your last remaining bit of patience; you have tried and tried to get your three-year-old child to accept one healthy food choice. This is a child who refuses to eat almost anything other than toast and the occasional piece of fruit. One night, you inform her that she will have to put her favorite toy away if she doesn't eat her dinner. She cries. You point to dinner and tell her that all she has to do is eat. She still refuses to eat, now so upset she probably couldn't eat even if she wanted to.

Finally, you feel like you are forced to follow through, and you set the beloved toy high on a shelf, telling your child that she can have it back the next morning. She learns quickly that she'll always get her toy back the next day, so at dinnertime the child simply tells her parent to go ahead and put the toy on the shelf. But she still doesn't eat. We teach, they learn, and they learn fast!

Why we do it

Because we're human. We are not provided an instruction manual when we become parents. In many cases, we feel we have tried everything else to get our child to eat. In some cases, threats might work to the extent that your child will eat a bite or two in order to escape the punishment, but ultimately this has not taught the child to be a healthy eater and has only added another dimension to the power struggle, elevating your level of frustration. No one wins.

Why it doesn't work

Threats damage a child's self-esteem and send the message that you don't have faith in your child to make the right decisions. "Threats are a message of distrust," says Adele Faber, author of *How to Talk So Kids Will Listen & How to Listen So Kids Will Talk.* "Your child hears, 'You can't be trusted to control yourself, so I'm going to control you.'"

The other problem with threats is that the parent has to be willing to follow through on the prescribed consequence. In the example above, the parent didn't enjoy taking the child's favorite toy away and was hoping that she wouldn't have to. In the virtuosity of good parenting, if you make a threat, you must be willing to live with the consequence for both you and your child. With food issues in particular, the punishment just doesn't fit the crime. It is not a natural consequence to remove a child's participation in a playmate's birthday celebration if he doesn't eat his peas, and this only teaches him that eating is something that is enforced superficially, and the child soon adapts to gain another level of control. Sounds like a cycle of coaching dysfunction.

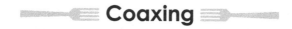

Coaxing

What it looks like

"Buzzzzz . . . here comes the airplane, open up the hangar."

Coaxing is something we have all participated in to encourage our children to eat. This is the kinder, gentler approach of trying to win a food fight. By using a friendly voice to appeal to our toddler's reasonable side, we try to convince him to eat, saying things like "Oh, my goodness! Don't those carrots look so delicious? Mommy's going to have some. Do you want some, too? No? Are you sure? They're so good." The airplane and other food games also fall under the coaxing category: "Open your mouth, T-Rex, here comes a bite of Stegosaurus!

Why we do it

In some ways, coaxing just seems natural. As parents, we do it all the time and it's a more positive approach than threatening or bribing. We think that by making a game out of eating and not allowing frustration to take over, we might ultimately get our child to eat. But with regard to eating, coaxing is still a scheming tool, no matter how nice we're being; it does not allow the child to learn a positive, well-balanced approach to taking control of eating behaviors.

Why it doesn't work

Coaxing, like threats and bribes, might work for some people some of the time. In a sense, the child might try something new to entertain the parent or get caught up in the game that they're playing—a role the parent expects them to play. Again, this might placate the parent's immediate concern of getting food into his child's belly, but does this slant really help to develop a healthy attitude about eating?

Another drawback is that the meal table ends up becoming a circus, complete with a frantic, anxious parent acting as the headlining entertainer during the evening show as he makes silly faces and turns food into flying spaceships. The applause and excitement of the other family members is designed to make the situation better because they want to be reassuring when the toddler finally eats something.

Nonetheless, this sets up a condition where the child is the absolute center of the family's attention, and the child will come to expect and desire this every night. It's simply too draining to keep up, and most parents become frustrated and eventually get to a point where they mutter, "I just want my child to eat," and they usually mean "without the additional hoopla." Not to mention the negative impact this can have on siblings who might not feel they are the center of their parents' attention. Which, I might add, can lead to a sibling-rivalry condition, and do you really need more to do? Then there is always the possibly of your other child or children engaging in the same actions, denying foods to gain more personalized parental attention. Save yourself the supplementary work. Don't do it.

Disguising Foods

What it looks like

"He'll never notice the pureed cauliflower I stuffed into his mashed potatoes."

Many ingenious parents come up with ways to hide nutritious foods in the not-so-nutritious foods their toddler essentially prefers. This is especially customary with vegetables, which are infamous for being less desirable to a picky eater. Although it is very common and perfectly acceptable to boost your soups and stews with as many vegetables or umami flavors as you can, this kind of food camouflage leads to a moral decision on the parent's part concerning whether to lie about it or not.

Why we do it

Parents are concerned about whether the child is getting enough of the vitamins and nutrition required from certain foods and worried about their child's vegetable intake. These qualms are addressed in Chapter Five.

Why it doesn't work

While it makes sense to pack as much nutrition as possible into our toddler's food, the long-term, complex portion of this deed is the moral dilemma of lying about it.

Despite a parent's best efforts, some children will notice the peas sticking out of their burger patty or the bitter taste of turnip processed into the mashed potatoes. For picky eaters, this camouflage practice can have the opposite effect from what the parents hoped. The picky eater may decline foods she had previously accepted once she realizes that the foods have been misrepresented. Now the child fears that she will find unfamiliar and objectionable foods hidden in the dinner she used to like. The child, who is essentially at the clemency of the parent feeding her, may then feel that she can't trust the parent and could become especially suspicious of trying new things.

Double-dealing your child about food, or anything for that matter, is not respectable practice. This parenting scheme can set up relationship issues later when an open line of communication is needed most—during tween and teen years. You can thank me later. Being honest about food or anything else at this age can help your child trust you, leading to a positive, open and engaged avenue of interaction later.

The One Bite Rule

What it looks like

"Just have one bite, and you don't have to eat anymore."
Very often the one bite rule is paired with a bribe: "Just have

one bite, and then you can go play with your friends." Often, parents establish the rule that every new food must be tried at least once. The one bite rule usually comes with a threat, such as the child not being allowed to leave the table until she has one more bite of broccoli.

Why we do it

Used in association with bribes and threats, the one bite rule works well for some parents, and they successfully manage to get their kids to eat an adequate portion of their meal. Likewise, some parents see it as a way to get youngsters to try new foods. If the obstinate toddler flatly refuses to take a bite of a green food, how will he know how good it is? Parents of picky eaters are always hopeful that their child will develop a liking for a new food, and the only way to accomplish that is for the child to try the food.

Why it doesn't work

While it seems like an innovative way to get a fussy child to try a new food, it is deeply rooted in the belief that the child will simply never try it on his own. Parents who practice the one bite rule feel that their child is incapable of proclaiming her own independence through trying new foods and that her apprehension will keep her from trying something new. While it might seem like your child will never try new foods, when the power struggle is taken out of the equation, your child will eventually become interested on her own and start exploring new foods. There are advanced food fight techniques ahead.

What happens when we lose the food fight?

Many despairing parents are guilty of turning their kitchens into all-day diners when all other efforts collapse. Some parents might prepare roast turkey with sweet potatoes for the whole family and then make chicken noodle soup with no noodles and a peanut butter sandwich with no jam for their picky eater. They might do it every night, no matter how tired they are or how little they feel like making special meals.

Although it may feel like your selflessness is serving a purpose, it's actually perpetuating an endless sequence in which your toddler is not encouraged to try new foods. The message you should be sending is that you trust your child to expand his food prospects. You don't want the child to think that he is "special" or "different" and therefore incapable of eating what everybody else is eating. This is a recipe for misfortune.

Parents, this is a relearn for us too. Try letting go of many of your peculiar food issues. Strive to become a little more relaxed. Maybe it is an issue surrounding cleanliness or always having to clean the plate from any waste. Whatever it is, avoid the power struggles and focus on relishing the special social interaction that mealtimes should provide. You might find your child exploring new foods at her own pace and in her own way.

Chapter Three

FOOD FIGHT STRATEGIES FOR CHILDREN

Ages Seven to Ten

While what-not-to-do techniques also work for this age range, you must also employ more maneuverability with the older age ranges, for obvious reasons. Different ages require different solutions based on developmental indicators. Children ages seven to ten will unquestionably need a higher calorie day. Make sure there are plenty of accessible foods left out in locations they frequent, e.g., the homework area, kitchen table, or reading area. Making healthy snack foods available for older kids when they return home from school or activities will make them more likely to grab some on the way to their next task. Make sure to keep this offering out for a short window of time so they don't fill up and not eat at a regularly-scheduled mealtimes.

Use the kitchen table as the primary location to sit and enjoy a snack. If the child does homework elsewhere, leave out a small portion of fresh-cut fruits and vegetables accompanying whole grain crackers and cheese. Set out dips and spreads such as homemade ranch, honey mustard, peanut spread or fresh yogurt with the addition of fresh herbs and flavored cream cheeses.

If kids are in between activities, such as sports or a club, this will help them replenish before heading on to the next great venture. Let them graze. Do not peddle the food.

As snacking behaviors introduced early are carried throughout teen years, dietary assessments should be carefully addressed at all ages and case by case. Every child is unique and will have diverse dietary needs. Keep in mind, it's widely accepted that younger children need to snack regularly. Kids ages three to seven have smaller stomach capacities and high nutrient requirements for growth and development. As children grow a bit older, parents must standardize the snacking before it leads to overconsumption. This doesn't mean to stop snacking, as it is important for total daily energy intake, but dietary interventions in children of all ages should be carefully balanced, and overserving should always be taken into account. A child's main meal strategies and activities should also be surveyed while balancing snacking. Research suggests that a higher number of snacking occasions is not associated with a higher body mass index (BMI) average, and suggests that snacking contributes to a positive energy uptake but should be monitored nonetheless.

Sample Snack-Time Suggestions

- Apple balls rolled in nut butter and granola
- Apples (red and green) cored and sliced. Never purchase pre-sliced and packaged apples—they are laden with chemicals to control browning. See Chapter Six for more information on processed foods.
- Sliced apple buffet with healthy dips
- Avocado boats (a quarter of an avocado) with pita chips
- Frozen banana rounds dipped in yogurt, or a side of yogurt dip

- Barely steamed or, better yet, raw broccoli florets. If steamed, quickly plunge in ice water to stop cooking. This professional chef technique will help you avoid the perpetual soggy broccoli problem and retain vibrant color and nutrients in all your vegetables.

- Cucumber sticks, skin on or off. I prefer to use seedless cucumber variety.

- Carrot coins or sticks or carrot paper (extremely-thin-sliced carrots). You can actually use a vegetable peeler and then place the carrot ribbons in ice water so they curl. I love adding these to my salads for fun.

- Cheese sticks, blocks, wedges or miniature cubes

- Chicken salad and crackers

- Warm, salted edamame

- Frozen peas. Try to introduce frozen peas for snacking (my kids loved snacking on these).

- Frozen grapes (not for small children under age seven—this is a choking hazard)

- Green Monster bombs

- Green pea guacamole

- Homemade fruit leathers

- Homemade mini empanadas

- Homemade pot stickers

- Homemade chicken nuggets

- Homemade fish fingers

- Lettuce wraps with your child's favorite fillings

- Mashed sweet potatoes, parsnips or garlic potatoes in a disposable pastry bag found at your local craft or baking store. Kids love the novelty of squeezing food into their mouths.

- Mini rice cakes with nut butters

- Muffins with tasty flavored compound butters
- Peanut butter popcorn
- Rice cake with nut butter and sliced pears or apples
- Smoothies with fruit and greens
- Spring roll wraps

Adding Dips or Toppings

Young children think that submerging foods in anything like dip is pure fun and delightfully messy. Older kids begin to evaluate the groupings of flavors and textures; best of all, they like the accessibility and independence to choose. This is a good opportunity to begin using closed-ended choices, a parenting practice I often used to manage my family.

Example: Offer two dips to choose from. Only two. This forces the child to choose within a controlled environment but allows the child to preserve her power through selecting one of them.

While offering closed-ended choices with a variety of foods, be sure to alternate selections until you find the one they love; then be prepared for change just when you are getting comfortable implementing a regular routine.

Add something different to the snack platter weekly. Trying new foods with older kids works especially well with afterschool snack time, when they are exceptionally hungry. If they don't eat it, at least they will look at it. Don't give up. Picky eaters will soon become familiar with the new foods placed on the snack platter. Don't discuss the new foods unless they ask, and if they do ask, respond matter-of-factly. Do not go into detail or spend time urging them to try the new food. They will look at it. This is actually one of the steps inside my advanced battle techniques. An important step for a picky eater is to visually identify the food before he touches it. If he doesn't touch it, that's fine. Wrap it up and put it away until the next snack platter.

Examples of Dips and Toppings

- Avocado yogurt puree
- Aioli
- Blue cheese
- Carrot yogurt
- Cauliflower puree
- Cream cheese, plain or flavored
- Compound butters
- Cucumber tzatziki
- Chopped dried fruit bits
- Edamame, warm with sea salt
- Freeze-dried banana chips
- Fruit coulis or homemade applesauce
- Fruit juices
- Guacamole with bread sticks or baked pita or stone-ground tortilla chips
- Green pea hummus
- Green goddess dressing
- Homemade ranch dip
- Italian dressing
- Low-fat cottage cheese (also great in baked potato skins or salted baked potato wedges; add a few topping choices to the tray for children to add on top of the potato skin themselves—this helps with power and control)
- Melted cheese pots
- Nutella (limited due to sugar content)
- Nuts and seeds
- Oils and vinegars (healthy oils such as extra virgin olive oil, avocado oil or coconut oil, and sweet rice vinegar or

    organic apple cider vinegar combined)

- Pasta sauce (warm or cold)
- Peanut or almond butters
- Peanut sauce
- Peanut butter and spun honey dip
- Pickle juice (As crazy as it sounds, some kids love it.)
- Pumpkin hummus
- Pureed fruits or vegetables
- Raisins or currents
- Ricotta cheese, plain or flavored
- Seven-layer bean dip
- Soy or ginger miso
- Trail mix
- Traditional hummus
- Tofu
- White bean dip
- Yogurt, plain or sweetened with natural juice or the addition of mild fresh herbs such as chervil, spices like garlic, or quick flavorings such as onion powder or salt. Or umami flavoring like mushroom powder, a few drops of Worcestershire, or fish sauce (sounds crazy, I know—don't worry; it won't taste like fish).

Building a Healthy Diet

Although healthy fats such as avocado, coconut oil, olive oil, organic butter, mayonnaise, and some dressings are not listed as part of a daily meal pattern, moderate amounts should be included daily. Healthy fats provide essential fatty acids, vitamin E, and they improve the palatability of meals and aid satiety in everyone. With regard to grain foods that are high in added sugars or anything highly processed in the market, consider not serving them at all. If you already began a particular unwholesome snack-time regime on a regular basis, set an initial limit, offering the food only two times per week; after a few weeks, restrict this offering to one time per week, and commit to a final date for completely weaning your child off the food in question.

When offering beverages and food at snack time, try to choose products that are lower in sodium. If it comes down to serving premade avocado dip versus smashing and seasoning your own avocado, consider not serving the premade-empty calorie food completely. Read the ingredient label of the avocado, salt and pepper, and compare these to the ingredient label of the pre-smashed avocado dip. Then make a choice. We should not be feeding our children artificial ingredients, especially children lacking in healthy eating patterns.

If you already set an unhealthy overall food regime or feed fast food every day, set an initial limit to ration these foods, serving them only three time per week, then twice per week, and soon once per week. Set a final date on your calendar for achieving the goal of diminishing the food in question completely. Two to three weeks into your goal, work toward completely weaning your child off the unhealthy food offering. Stay firm.

If your family or child can tolerate wheat or grain products and you are currently using stripped, hulled wheat or grain products such as faster cooking rice or oats, keep your regime going until you find an acceptable product that aligns with foods containing whole grain content. Work toward changing to whole grain products completely. Today, whole grains are mainstream and have become more available and affordable, not to mention varied. Some families will also change the feed times to contain whole grain-rich-foods or increase their proportion in a certain meal or snack times to meet required daily uptakes.

Children from six or seven years up begin to participate in a wide range of sports and might require more calories from carbohydrate sources. Remember, each child's energy needs are different. For instance, your child may need more energy during growth spurts or active participation in sports. It's not necessary to eat the exact total amounts from each group every day. Rather, intake should average out over a period of one to two weeks to ensure healthy intake of calories along with essential nutrients.

The US Department of Agriculture (USDA) recommends daily calorie values for each age group, as summarized in Chapter One.[1] These are only guidelines. Children should not be on restricted calories unless under a doctor's supervision. Keep in mind that if your child consumes extra calories beyond what is needed, the calories need to be burned off with extra physical activity or he could be on the road to obesity. Extra empty calories can quickly add up depending on what your children eat or drink. If your child eats or drinks an extra 100 calories each day beyond his or her caloric need and does not burn off the extra calories, that's an extra 700 calories each week, an extra 2,800 each month, and an extra 36,500 calories each year. If you have to choose which mealtime to shave an unhealthy calorie from, start the day out right by supplying closed-ended choices first thing in the morning; choose healthy foods to your child's liking. Eating breakfast helps your child start his day in a healthy way. Integrate fruit and whole grains whenever possible. Children and adults who eat breakfast daily are less likely to be overweight.[2]

As parents, we can help our youngsters make the right nutrition choices from a primary age. Do this by engaging your child in a few activities when it comes to food choices. This age range can decide what and how much to eat, under mild supervision, of course. Empower his choices and decisions with positive reinforcement. Control the food groups by giving him two healthy choices to choose from, like an apple and an orange. The child still gains power and control, but within a boundary you supply. It's a great way for your kids to get excited about eating healthy foods. Let them decide what and how much to eat.

Allow your children to help you with small, child-safe jobs in the kitchen, such as mixing ingredients and setting the table. Allow them to smell, touch, taste, and play with the food. Talk

---

1   See Dietary Guidelines for Americans for additional guidance; calories from protein, carbohydrates, and total fats should be within the acceptable macronutrient distribution ranges (AMDRs). Values are rounded. Available at www.cnpp.usda.gov/USDAFoodPatterns

2   Stephen J. Pont, Rebecca Puhl, Stephen R. Cook, Wendelin Slusser, "Stigma Experienced by Children and Adolescents with Obesity," *Pediatrics*, November 2017.

about the colors, where they came from, how they were grown. Is the food from the soil or a tree? Note the color variety and talk about its history if you know it. Bring up the nutrition value and why we eat it. Not all children will be curious, but some will. Not everyone will eat foods they prepare, but preparing will pique interest in it. Don't force it to happen. Touching foods they would normally not consume is a very good first step.

Chapter Four

CREATING GOOD EATING HABITS | IDENTIFYING FOOD INTOLERANCES

We can't force our kids to eat, but we can be role models regarding what and when to eat. One of the most powerful ways to teach a child anything is to model the kind of behavior you want to see them emulate. If you want your children to become adults who enjoy a wide variety of nutritious foods, make sure you eat the foods you'd like them to eat. If healthy eating is a way of life in your home, it is likely your children will grow up to follow the same habits. Also, if they grow up experiencing regular mealtimes, there's a good chance they will continue that pattern.

Childhood's impulse to imitate is strong. Your youngster will watch what you're eating, so make sure your plate is always filled with healthy selections. If you're asking your child to eat vegetables and fish while you graze on potato chips and soda, your illustration will override your good intentions. Remember, parenting by example will help you set boundaries and make follow-through easier; something as simple as eating healthy will be your best course of action.

Serving Sizes

Ever really wonder how many servings of vegetables a toddler needs? How much milk she should drink from a bottle or a cup? There are so many questions we have as parents, and while we are faced with the greatest and most important job on the planet, the job comes without a training manual. In the age of technology and the internet, we are also faced with the fact that some information we seek off the World Wide Web could be incorrect. If you do seek any information via the internet regarding your child's nutrition values, make sure it is coming from a reputable source. And always consult your healthcare provider first.

Most children should be offered three to five servings of vegetables a day, but for children under five, each serving only needs to be a tablespoon for each year of age. Yes, it's that easy. In other words, a two-year-old should ideally consume two tablespoons of vegetables three to five times a day. So, if you are not the proud parent of a veggie lover, try a few of my fun food fight activities, listed in Chapter Eight. How much food a child needs to feel full can really only be determined by the child. It is important early on to acknowledge and respect a child's signs of hunger and satiety so that the child can learn to trust these instincts and eat accordingly. This is why it is so crucial for parents to understand that their role is to provide a variety of foods at meal and snack times, and it is their child's role to decide how much he will eat. Sometimes parents' expectancies are excessive due to our distorted vision of what a portion size is. Become familiar with toddler-size portions. An effective rule of thumb is: one tablespoon per year of age = one portion.[3] Example: One tablespoon of peas is a serving for a one-year-old.

---

3   American Academy of Pediatrics, *Your Child's Nutrition: Making Peace at the Table and Building Healthy Eating Habits for Life* (New York: Villard Books, 1999).

Making Snacks Simple and Fun

Make simple, appetizing snacks exciting by placing them in a fun arrangement or playful containers. Try placing snacks in an ice cube tray, or egg cartons, or in a rainbow design on a big platter. Designing shapes is fun. But don't become a short-order cook. If you have time for fun arrangements, that's great. If you don't, that's okay too—fancy is not required. A plate is just as good. We also don't want our children to get in the habit of expecting these magnificent arrangements from us on a regular basis. I'm not saying to pass up the opportunity to engage in magic childhood fun, but don't make such a habit of it that a picky eater uses this as a reason not to eat.

Serve a rainbow of colors to ensure a full offering of nutrients daily. You can also invite the child to participate in the shopping and preparation of foods in your kitchen, giving him small tasks such as washing, peeling, mixing, and arranging food on a plate. Be sure to talk about the color of the foods and the benefits to eating them without sounding like you are trying to drive him to eat it. Be natural and move onto the next subject. Don't wait for an acknowledgement or a response. Just provide a matter-of-fact commentary about the food you are preparing at the moment. If the children help in the kitchen, make sure they understand ahead of time that they need to also be involved in the cleanup. Add fruits and veggies to foods your child already enjoys; nudge blueberries into pancakes, or dice fruit and pop it onto wholesome cereal. If your child does not have a fixation on foods touching or colors blending, pop a few small pieces of cooked peas or broccoli on your homemade macaroni and cheese.

Avoiding Food Traps

What are food traps? Well, we all have been tangled up in them at one time or another. Food traps are situations that make it difficult for us to eat healthy or feed our families healthy. Especially picky eaters. When parents are faced with a picky eater, every bite counts; getting ourselves and our family caught up in a food trap just creates another obstacle to providing healthy and nutritious choices. Once this happens, we begin to see changes such as not eating on time, skipping meals, or giving into fast food options. Some examples of food traps are road trips, holidays, playgroup meet-ups, family vacations, and difficulty with time management. Even other family members can make things more difficult when it comes to feeding our own families.

If traveling, pack healthy snacks your picky eater will agree to. Make sure you avoid fast foods; if you choose to stop at a casual dining restaurant, choose wisely. Traveling by car, we can be inundated with fast food road signs everywhere. Voice your fast food rules before the trip.

When it's time for family celebrations outside your immediate family and, quite possibly, an end-of-the-year holiday gathering, go ahead and celebrate—just don't lose sight of what and when your child is eating. Make sure to educate and not send a feeling of negativity about eating a celebratory cookie or portion of cake you wouldn't normally allow your child to indulge in, and then ensure your child eats a balanced meal.

Soda during celebrations? Make sure you portion control. Not only because it is an empty calorie, but also because you should take into consideration whether your child is accustomed to consuming trans fats, sugars, or artificial ingredients; she could have a slight reaction. Everything in moderation, right?

Involved in a playgroup? Worried about empty calorie foods there? Bring a fruit or veggie tray to share. Make a closed-ended choice quietly with your child. Maybe she chooses to indulge and also eat a healthy snack. Don't force it or announce it—simply gauge it, especially in a social setting. If there is another child eating healthy, place your child next to that child. Don't point out or call out. Your child will naturally observe her peers. Sometimes during playtime, kids are so wound up they won't eat—that's okay too. This just primes their evening appetite. Could be a win-win for us. Hungry children eat.

I also believe it is just as important to not talk about our food choices as it is to talk about them. Confusing, right? Well, it really comes down to when and where we have these discussions and how long we discuss. As parents, we are not in the business to frighten our children to the point they cannot function as they grow. Unfortunately, food shaming or exploiting can leave negative results on a child later in life. Our choices on how we present to our children should be enacted with moderation.

I've seen some instances where parents are so neurotic about food choices that their children grow up unable to manage normality surrounding food. Other parents unintentionally create an outcast-type environment among their children's peers by overexerting food choices for their child. This is often noticeable at school and in after-school groups or group activities, where some children feel they have been selected or tagged within a social circle. Some of this is due to the parents' expectations of their child's food choices, which can be easily exasperated by society and even other parents. This is especially difficult for children living with food intolerances and growing into the already challenging preteen years.

An over-responsive parent may create additional pressure. Go easy and lead with moderation. If your child has a food intolerance, work specifically with your child; just don't expect other parents to change how they feed their children for you— they might overcompensate to show support and unknowingly label your child among the group. This can open a variety of social issues for your child later.

Parents of preteens and tweens, please don't embarrass your children publicly. Discuss their food intolerances with them privately. There is also no need to tell the whole school, other parents, and the administration that your child is dealing with a food challenge. Empower your child; teach her to know the better choice for her without becoming that overbearing, neurotic parent.

The other side of the coin: If your child does suffer from food intolerances, you will see a physical reaction, which should be taken very seriously. A recent study from the American Pediatrics Association reported that over 30 percent of children with food allergies say they have been bullied about their allergies. Previous studies also found that having a food allergy can put a child at risk for bullying.

[4]Food sharing is one of the most basic social constants in human culture. We use food as our social binding. When a group shares food, we are saying we are a community. Many cultural traditions and religious rituals involve the sharing of food. Some psychologists agree that humans also use food as a way of increasing status within the group. We use food as a way of connecting with one another. So, what is the significance when an individual cannot participate in these basic social interfaces? Asking this question can help us understand the social stigma of food allergies or intolerances. Look at the same situation from the perspective of a child with a parent who obsesses over the picky eater's food choices.

We all know the scenario. Whenever cupcakes were brought to class, a classmate, or maybe your child, was not able to eat one. Yes, someone, maybe yourself, provided him with some other treat, but the deeper message was that he could not share what the others were eating and was not part of the group. Every event based on food sharing becomes a reminder of his separateness. The cupcake is a reminder that the adults in charge did not think he was important enough to be included. The situation could also draw too much attention to said child. I feel the same when I am on a chosen nutrition regime. Going out to dinner with friends or any group activity surrounded by food seems to illuminate my personal choice, and everyone seems to think they need to discuss it. It's amazing. As an adult, I can compartmentalize and rationalize what is happening, but as a child things like this can leave an impression, good or bad to be determined, and are you willing to wait and see?

An easy example of the kind of food-sharing interaction we all take for granted: A parent brings cupcakes to class. Each student is offered a cupcake and enjoys the sweet treat. The students' trust and liking for this parent is increased.

The birthday student is a celebrity for a day, and when the other kids have their birthdays, they ask their parents to bring cupcakes. What happens when there is a student with a food allergy or intolerance in the class? Your child is offered a cupcake,

---

4   Stevens JR, Gilby IC. A conceptual framework for nonkin food sharing: timing and currency of benefits. Animal Behavior 2009

but he must say, "No thank you, I have food allergies." He is allergic to egg, and these cupcakes almost certainly contain egg.

This is the first moment where the food-sharing ritual breaks down. The food-sensitive person is forced to refuse the offer of food. In many cultures, refusing an offer of food is considered rude. Even though he gives the reason (food allergies), this is often not accepted. People become defensive and don't believe that the allergy is real or serious. They offer objections: Their friend's child is allergic to egg but can tolerate baked goods, so this cupcake is okay; "A little bit won't hurt"; they are "pretty sure" the item doesn't contain eggs, and so on. To them, his rejection of the food feels like a rejection of the person offering it. Same conditions can apply if a parent is too obsessive over feed times. Identify the patterns you create in discussions with your picky eater, and try to work on bringing these discussions to a minimum in public. Do not overdo it.

Of course, picky and selective eating is different from a dangerous food allergy or a food intolerance; however, my point is to be aware how we, as parents, can change the social landscape of our children by over-discussing within peer groups. Don't make it a big deal, and you might have less of an issue to deal with down the road.

Keep in mind that some picky eaters are naturally picky because they are having a physical negative reaction that you may be unaware of. If your child is not able to verbally tell you, again, look for cues. There are all sorts of reasons your child is a picky eater. If the food is bothering your child, it's time to talk to your health care provider. Don't wait.

Identifying Food Intolerances

Food intolerance is a gastrointestinal system response rather than an immune system response. Food intolerance occurs when something in your child's food irritates her digestive system. Your child's gastric system might be unable to break down food properly, and as a result your child may get a bellyache, cramps, bloating, and headaches. A good sign to watch for is your child becoming irritable.

A food allergy, on the other hand, is an immune system response. It is caused when your child's body mistakes an ingredient in food, often a casein protein, as harmful and creates a defense system to fight it. An allergic reaction can affect the whole body, not just digestion. Symptoms may include a rash, hives, itchy skin, shortness of breath, chest pain, a sudden drop in blood pressure, and trouble swallowing or breathing.

Unfortunately, most food intolerances are found through trial and error. Your child's pediatrician or nutrition specialist may ask you to keep a food diary for several weeks and record everything your child eats. When the child experiences symptoms, this should also be noted, especially the type of discomfort the child is experiencing. This information will assist your healthcare provider to identify any underlying, common factors that might indicate food intolerances.

Another way to identify problematic foods is through an elimination diet. You would begin by completely eliminating any suspect foods from your child's diet until he is symptom-free. This takes some time. It is important to stay vigilant and patient. After eliminations, you then reintroduce the foods one at a time, which can help pinpoint which foods are causing the symptoms. You must seek the advice of your doctor or specialist before beginning an elimination diet to ensure your child is still receiving adequate nutrition. If your child has food intolerance, symptoms usually appear gradually; they might only appear when your child eats a lot of a certain food or eats something often. Food intolerances are usually not life threatening, but there are some foods that can cause an anaphylactic response, which could be fatal if not attended to quickly. Food allergies are much more likely to come on suddenly and be triggered by even the smallest amount of food. This is likely to happen every time your child eats a particular food and can be life threatening depending on the level of response and severity of the symptoms.

Picky eaters are struggling with power and control. They will not show signs of food intolerances or food allergies, but they will still reduce food intake. Usually these refusals are accompanied with crying or tantrums and followed by eating something they pushed you into preparing.

Common food intolerances include:

- Dairy
- Eggs
- Gluten—the protein in wheat, rye, oats and barley
- Sugar—particularly if your child has candida, a yeast overgrowth that can affect behavior and is very common in children with neurobehavioral challenges such as ADHD and autism.
- Shellfish
- Soy
- Foods high in salicylate—salt or ester of a salicylic acid
- Food dyes
- Preservatives, artificial ingredients
- Pesticides
- Some GMOs—genetically modified foods

The link between diet and behavior is an interesting one, especially when food sensitivities are involved.

Chapter Five

HEALTHY GUIDELINES

T he USDA food configurations were developed to help individuals carry out dietary guideline recommendations; they identify daily amounts of foods, in nutrient-dense forms, to eat from five major food groups and their subgroups.[5] The patterns also include an allowance for oils and a limit on the maximum number of calories available for other uses, such as added sugars, solid fats, and added refined starches. I've outlined suggestions for age-range subgroups throughout this chapter and in future chapters.

---

5   Daniel J. Raiten, Ramkripa Raghavan, Alexandra Porter, Julie E. Obbagy, and Joanne M. Spahn, "Executive summary: Evaluating the evidence base to support the inclusion of infants and children from birth to 24 mo of age in the Dietary Guidelines for Americans—'the B-24 Project,'" The American Journal of Clinical Nutrition (March 2014): 663-691.

Sample Portions for a Typical Two-to-Five-Year-Old

Grains
- 1/2–1 slice of bread
- 1/2–3/4 cup of cereal
- 1/2–1 small muffin
- 1/2 cup of rice or pasta

Vegetables and Fruit
- 1/2–1 medium vegetable or fruit
- 1/4–1/2 cup of frozen, canned, or fresh fruit or vegetables (Avoid canned foods if possible.)
- 1/2–1 cup of salad
- 1/4–1/2 cup of juice

Dairy
- 1–2 ounces of cheese
- 1/2–3/4 cup of yogurt
- 1/2–1 cup of milk

Animal Proteins and Alternatives
- 1–2 ounces of meat, fish or poultry
- 1 egg
- 1/4–1/2 cup of beans
- 1/4–1/3 cup of tofu
- 1–2 tablespoons of nut butters

Sample Menus

Breakfast
- 1/2 cup of cereal with 1/2 cup of milk
- 1/2 cup of juice

Mid-Morning Snack
- 1/2 cup of yogurt with 1/4 cup of berries

Lunch
- 1/4 grilled cheese sandwich
- 2–3 carrot coins with dip
- 1/2 cup of milk

Afternoon Snack
- 1/2 a piece of toast with 1 tablespoon of peanut butter
- 1/2 cup of goat, cow, soy, almond, or rice milk beverage
- 1/2 apple or banana

Dinner
- 1/2 cup of noodles with 2 tablespoons of pasta sauce
- 1 tablespoon of frozen peas
- 1/2 meatball

Dessert
- 1/2 cup of yogurt
- 1/2 apple

Snack
- 1/2 cup of nut, goat, or cow milk
- 2 crackers

Remember to respect tiny tummies and tongues. Keep food servings small. Wondering how much to offer? Here's a rule of thumb—or rather, of hand: A young child's stomach is approximately the size of her fist; dole out small portions at first and refill the plate if your child asks for more. This less-is-more meal plan not only is more successful with picky eaters, it also has the added benefit of stabilizing blood sugar levels, which in turn decreases mood swings. Touch and texture round out the senses, too.

Spicy foods taste "hot" and trigger pain fibers in the mouth, which makes most kids reject them. Some children are very sensitive to certain textures of food, which can often be a larger reason they won't like the taste. Keep in mind that food can be different to children than adults. What you taste might not be what they taste.

How to Be Successful with Closed-Ended Choices

Lifelong health begins in infancy, yet all too soon our kids are barraged by messages that thwart our efforts. Between peer pressure and television commercials advertising junk foods, getting children to eat well might seem more futile than fruitful. So, what exactly can parents do to instill healthy eating habits in their kids?

You can make a huge impression on your child's lifelong relationship with food through simple things like getting kids involved in food preparation, focusing on the food, and sharing time with family. Parents should always model positive actions around food and nutrition with your own healthy choices and gestures. A really great mealtime strategy is simply turning off the television and engaging in a conversation about the day. I would begin these conversations by asking my child, "What was the best thing that happened to you today?" Followed by, "What was the worse?" You would be surprised what you can learn. And this is what the family mealtime table should be doing: engaging everyone in positive, feel-good participation. Your child will feel an added benefit of expression, accompanied by some relief that you're not so focused on the policy of food choices.

The challenge facing the parent of a picky eater is to make healthy choices appealing. And it is work. No matter how good your intentions are, trying to convince your eight-year-old that an apple is as sweet a treat as a chocolate-dipped cookie won't work. Be transparent and honest. And remember, it's perfectly okay to not talk about the chocolate-dipped cookie. You are in control or aspiring to be. Ensure that your child's diet is as nutritious and wholesome as possible, even while allowing for some of his favorite treats. You can please both your child's palate and your sense of parental responsibility by using positive parenting campaigns. One that worked for my family over and over was offering a closed-ended choice. I found this technique shared by a few of my favorite parenting experts: [6]Adele Faber and Elaine Mazlish. They educated me through their books and parenting workshops on how closed-ended choices allow children to feel empowered to make a choice, which makes the children feel in control; however, your role is to control the options. Offer a choice between two items only, and suggest the child choose one.

Example:

"You can choose an apricot or an orange for today's mid-morning snack." Then wait. Ask again, but with different content. "And did you want it peeled or cut into sections?"

Expected Outcome:

This technique of closed-ended choices can be very empowering for the both of you. When my children were little, I had difficulties with bathing time. Offering a bath with or without bubbles solved our power struggles, and fast. You can use this tactic with food and gain the same success—it just takes some practice.

---

6   Adele Faber, and Elaine Mazlish, *How to Talk So Kids Will Listen & Listen So Kids Will Talk* (New York: Scribner, 2012).

Simple Strategies for Toddlers

Offer Happy Hour

Toddlers like to graze their way through a variety of foods. Offer your child a customized smorgasbord. This is clearly an opportunity for closed-ended food offerings. Use an ice-cube tray, a muffin tin or a compartmentalized dish. Put bite-size portions of colorful and nutritious whole foods in each section. Give these finger foods playful names that a two-year-old can appreciate. Older toddlers will be just as happy with this, especially after preschool or group activities. Keep all grazing times synchronized with other mealtimes so they won't fill up and not eat at scheduled times. Example: Do not provide snacks 30 to 60 minutes before dinner.

Suggestions of whole foods include:

- Apple smiles (thinly-sliced apple wedges)
- Avocado pieces
- Frozen-yogurt-dipped banana coins
- Broccoli trees (gently steamed broccoli florets)
- Cucumber sticks with tangy yogurt dip (cucumbers cut lengthwise)
- Carrot ribbons or coins (raw or almost cooked through, and thinly sliced)
- Cheese blocks (cubes of cheese)
- Peas, frozen or thawed (I never offer canned or pre-prepared foods.)
- Mashed sweet potatoes on a whole wheat cracker

Make your life easier. When kids have a timed grazing period, it can equal good behavior. A child's demeanor often parallels her eating patterns. Parents might notice that a toddler's behavior deteriorates toward the end of the morning or mid-afternoon. Behavior continues to worsen the longer she goes without food. Timed grazing minimizes blood sugar swings and lessens the resulting undesirable mood swings. Grazing gives the child power to choose from an array of foods you have controlled. By offering a timed grazing period, you will create a silent closed-ended choice environment. The child feels somewhat satisfied, allowed to make choices within a boundary you have supplied.

To support grazing success, place the food choices on an easy-to-reach table. As your toddler makes her rounds through the house, she can stop, sit down, and nibble a bit inside the designated grazing area. When she's done chewing and swallowing she can continue on her way. Use foods that have a table-life of an hour or two. If you are worried about choking hazards, cut foods into small, manageable pieces, and offer a closed-ended choice on playing while grazing. Set the rules of location and time, and use the timer. Once the timer rings, pick the food up and do not re-feed until the following mealtime. Be consistent with these rules on all offered grazing times.

For instance, a child can only stay in the kitchen area while grazing and is not allowed to talk with food in the mouth due to a choking hazard. Tell your child why. Don't just say, "Don't talk with food in your mouth." Explain why we don't talk, walk or run while eating or drinking. Set the timer for a thirty to sixty minute period. She will also begin to identify with the sound of the timer. If she doesn't get the hang of the rules this time, you can bet she will learn soon. It will take a few times, but if you follow the rules yourself, this process will become predictable for your child, just like brushing teeth before bed or bath-time sequences. Once your child's body clock adjusts to snack time, you can stop using the timer.

Children will respond to how you present each food fight technique. Are you presenting this time period as an enjoyable period? Or are you placing pressure on the child by setting a negative tone? Are you using a "Let's see if *this* works" tone that will create a passive-aggressive feeling? If you have presented an activity negatively, your child will mirror the same negative tone or act out negatively.

Also consider that small children have no concept of time. Timed grazing activities can help them gain a consciousness surrounding your family schedule. Always provide a five to ten minute warning. If the timer will sound in five minutes, tell your child that you will be picking up the snacks in five minutes— or ten laps around the kitchen, which could be the equivalent to five minutes. Provide a depiction of something to help your toddler identify just how long a five-minute length of time is. Be fair but firm.

Chapter Six

DEVELOPING POSITIVE EATING HABITS EARLY

O besity among children has become endemic in North America. If children start to develop healthy eating habits at a young age, they will be much better off and may sidestep becoming part of these terrible statistics. If you've discovered that the only thing your child will eat is high-fat, processed fast food and you give in because it's better than nothing, the probability that he or she will become overweight is very likely. It's important to get into the habit of ensuring that the only food in the house is healthy food. It's very difficult to change habits established in childhood. As you explore your child's palate, also keep in mind that whether something looks good or "yucky" in a child's eyes greatly contributes to the flavor of the food. Kids, just like adults, eat with their eyes first. That's why a child might immediately like a pretty food found in an advertisement or menu. Marketing and media have a huge impact on children.

The Implications of Good Eating Habits

Good eating habits that are established when you're young are likely to stick with you for life. You're less prone to illness, and you're more likely to preserve a healthy weight, which might also have a positive impact on your self-worth. Positive self-worth affects every area of your life.

Trust Your Child's Instincts

Pediatricians often tell parents that they shouldn't worry—their picky toddler won't starve himself. Many parents are still concerned that their child isn't eating adequately. The truth is, children have remarkably good instincts when it comes to their food choices. When given the opportunity without power struggles (bribing, coaxing and threatening), they will eat exactly what their body needs. We just need to offer the right choices for them to cherry-pick from.

If you want your child to eat dinner at the same time you do, try to appropriately time his snacks at least two hours before dinner. Some children are fed snacks prior to mealtime and then punished for not eating. However, because their tummies are so small, they really are just full and not necessarily being picky.

When to Start Good Eating Habits

Now! Make every calorie count. Offer your child foods that pack lots of nourishment into small doses. This is particularly important for toddlers, who are often as active as rabbits yet seem to eat like mice.

Eating a lot of high-fat, processed convenience foods can become a habit because it's easy. If you don't start feeding your child processed foods in the first place, you won't have to break a difficult habit. Foods containing trans fats can coat the tongue, leaving taste buds unreceptive and hypnotizing us into preferring unhealthy flavors and food textures.[7] Again, if you can avoid processed foods, you should.

---

7   David Van Vranken, and Gregory Weiss, *Introduction to Bioorganic Chemistry and Chemical Biology* (New York: Garland Science, 2012).

Nutrient-Dense Foods Most Children Are Willing to Eat If Introduced Early

- Avocados
- Pasta
- Broccoli
- Peanut butter
- Brown rice and other whole grains
- Potatoes
- Cheese
- Poultry
- Eggs
- Squash
- Fish
- Sweet potatoes
- Kidney beans
- Tofu
- Yogurt
- Cucumbers

Count on Inconsistency

For young children, what and how much they are willing to eat may vary daily. Again, just be patient and remember that children will test boundaries while finding their role and place in the family structure. They are seeking independence, and eating is an area where they can feel an enormous sense of control.

Don't be surprised if your child eats a heaping plateful of food one day and practically nothing the next; adores broccoli on Tuesday and refuses it on Thursday; or wants to feed herself at one meal and be entirely dependent on you another time. As a parent or caregiver, it's up to you to provide a consistent blueprint for toddlers to flourish in. Stay patient though the inconsistency. Simplifying with healthy foods will assist your picky eater's mood swings; snacking choices in between meals will help with blood sugar spikes—and don't take the mood swings personally. Some parents get embarrassed when their child acts out, especially in public. Just tune everyone out. The world is full of judgments.

Don't stray from your job as a loving parent because of social pressure. Parenting is stressful, and it is easy to get really annoyed and say things we don't mean because we are so exhausted. Your job is the most important job in the entire world. Love your child and offer positive parenting whenever the opportunity to teach arises. It is a child's job to be a child. If he knew better than to throw himself on the floor and cry, he would be an adult; teach to that. Mark these words: One day, you will miss those annoying parental days.

We never know where the road will lead. Just follow the signs and anticipate your child's needs. My older children still express themselves in the same way. One week they are packing individual yogurts all week, so the following week I buy extra individual yogurts—and then they won't eat them. Nevertheless, I still offer closed-ended food choices by stocking the refrigerator and pantry with healthy food choices.

Fixation

Sometime between the second and third birthday, you can expect your child to become set in his ideas on just about everything, including the way food is prepared—expect food fixations. If the peanut butter must be on top of the jelly and you put the jelly on top of the peanut butter . . . be prepared for a protest. It's not easy to reason with an opinionated three-year-old. It is better to make the sandwich the child's way; don't interpret this as his being stubborn. Toddlers have a mindset about the order of things in their world. Any alternative is unacceptable. Don't worry. This is a passing stage and a rite of passage for all parents.

Chapter Seven

THE LIQUID DIET

Milk, the Child's Staple

Many parents offer their child milk throughout the day and feel that at least their picky eater is getting some nutrition. While this is true to some extent, offering milk is not the answer to your child's refusal to eat a variety of solid foods. In fact, if your child drinks too much milk, he can suffer deficiencies of important vitamins and minerals because he will be too full to eat other essential foods. The size of a toddler's stomach is very small and can be filled easily. If your two-year-old has asked for milk several times between breakfast and lunch and you have given it to her, she will be less likely to sit down and eat the peanut butter sandwich at lunchtime.

For younger toddlers who have been bottle-fed, it seems only natural to give them several cups or bottles of milk throughout the day. However, if your eighteen-month-old is at the stage and is ready and willing to try supplementary solid foods, then it might be time to start weaning him off bottles and limiting his milk consumption. Check with your child's doctor and ask how much milk your child should consume at his age and weight.

Milk vs. No Milk

It can be difficult for some parents to "let milk go" when milk was the child's main nutritional source for a very long time—either in formula or breast milk. However, once a child starts eating solid foods (around the age of one), solid food should become the main source of nutrition, and milk should become only a beverage.

How much milk is enough?

Toddlers need 500 mg of calcium a day and 200 international units (IU) of vitamin D.[8] The main reason pediatricians and nutritionists recommend milk in a toddler's diet is because one cup of milk has 300 mg of calcium and 98 IU of vitamin D, so if your child has two cups of milk a day, she is more than covered. However, some parents elect not to give their children cow's milk at all due to lactose allergies, personal taste, or concern about the hormones used in the production of milk. If you choose not to give your child cow's milk, there are other options, such as goat, fortified soy, rice and nut milks. Calcium-added orange juice has the same calcium content as cow's milk.

One point to note is that some brands of soymilk contain sugar, which can wreak havoc on developing teeth. Also, for older toddlers, it's better to serve drinks in cups and not bottles. Limit the use of sippy cups, which, while handy to prevent spills, make it easier for bacteria to hang around in your child's mouth when she sucks on the cup's spout. Check with your child's doctor and dentist. Finding a replacement for vitamin D can be tricky. Egg yolks and oily fish contain vitamin D. Furthermore, when your child gets plenty of outside time in the sun, his body produces its own. However, wintertime could pose a problem.

If you have decided not to serve your child milk, I have listed some calcium-rich food alternatives, but please check with your child's doctor.

---

8   Institute of Medicine, *Dietary Reference Intakes for Calcium and Vitamin D* (Washington, DC: The National Academies Press, 2010).

Calcium-Rich Food Alternatives to Milk:

- Breads
- Cheese of all types
- Cottage cheese
- Cooked dried beans
- Eggs
- Fruit
- Green leafy veggies
- Meat/poultry/fish
- Noodles
- Nuts and seeds
- Tofu
- Vegetables
- Yogurt (Watch for high sugar content.)

Hitting the Bottle

We all know toddlers love juice, and what's not to love? Even 100 percent juice with no added sugar, which is what your child should be drinking, is a sweet treat. However, the dangers of too much juice offset the benefits. Below are some reasons why giving your child too much juice will only cause problems in the long run.

Although it may seem like you're giving your child a healthy apple every time you hand over a cup of apple juice, it is actually much better to just cut up and serve the apple instead. The American Association of Pediatrics recommends that only 50 percent of the daily fruit requirement for toddlers and preschoolers should come from drinking juice.

Children under 6 months of age should not be offered juice. The American Association of Pediatrics recommends breastfeeding as the sole source of nutrition for your baby for about six months. When you add solid foods to your baby's diet, continue breastfeeding until at least twelve months if you can. If you cannot, that's okay too; at least you can say you tried. You can continue to breastfeed after twelve months if you and your baby desire. Check with your child's doctor about vitamin D and iron supplements during the first year.

Hold off feeding juice until twelve months of age. For children ages one to six, limit juice to 4 to 6 ounces per day. For children older than six years, fruit juice offers no nutritional benefits over whole fruits. Whole fruits also provide fiber and other nutrients.

Do not allow your child to carry a cup or box of juice throughout the day; this will just prompt your toddler to fill up on juice and not eat. Ages seven and up should limit juice to 8 ounces a day. The natural sugars in juice can cause tooth decay, which can be devastating for a young child, who must then spend hours in the dentist chair having cavities filled. Juice is especially hard on developing teeth if it's served in bottles; it should always be offered in a cup. Unfortunately, milk can have the same effect on developing teeth.

Always make sure you serve 100 percent real fruit juice to get the full nutritional value. Any juice that is described with the words *drink, cocktail* or *beverage* is usually made with ample amounts of sugar and not a lot of actual fruit juice. High fructose corn syrup is not a recommended healthy choice by the American Association of Pediatrics, and you should avoid any foods or drinks containing this product.

Don't be fooled by sports drinks. Read nutrition labels. If your child is playing a sport, water is a great refreshment and source of replenishment. Unless your child is exercising like a pro-athlete, she is not likely losing enough electrolytes to warrant a sports drink, and reliable food can replace any losses of sodium.

Be Your Own Arsenal

At this point, you should be fortified with enough knowledge to trust that your child will not starve or become malnourished from picky eating alone. This is usually the first step toward food fight freedom.

Keep in mind that toddlers and preschoolers are notoriously erratic with their eating habits and may not conform to the "daily recommended amounts" from the government-mandated food guides but rather plot out their nutritional intake on their own timetable. You provide. They will eat. But prepare to schedule changes as they age. Start to practice your own closed-ended choice sentences. This does take some practice. You will find yourself rewinding and starting over until you feel confident with your delivery. Just practice.

Chapter Eight

MAKING MEALTIMES FUN

Clearly the dinner table in your home is an endless battle zone or you would not be reading this. The fact is, the dinner table can either be a place for your family to come together peacefully, or it can try your patience. Our kids use food as a means of control. If we choose to engage in the struggle, we create a battle zone.

First things first: make sure baby is rested.

Toddlers have a difficult time sitting at the table for more than a minute or two. Often, it's best just to accept that they might not sit at the dinner table; if they do, don't insist they sit for the duration of the meal. Let them wander. When you let go and give yourself the time to enjoy your meal, you can be a better parent. Eating on the run or spending most of the time hopping up and down from the table trying to get a two-year-old to eat is not a reasonable pattern. As children get older, they're capable of sitting at the table for the duration of the meal, and by the time they reach school age, it's something we can insist on.

If your child doesn't want to eat what's in front of him, it is not your job to become a short-order cook, unless of course he has food allergies and requires a special diet. If you get into the habit of catering to special orders just to appease a fussy child, you set a precedent you're probably going to resent later on. If he likes what's presented, that's great, but if he doesn't, invite him to eat what he likes. You don't have to come across as punitive or judgmental.

If you insist that your kids eat everything on their plates and they've decided they're not going to, you're in for a very trying and challenging time. It's a battle, and you're likely going to lose. Disengage from these types of old-school expectations. The only thing they are good for is ruining relationships and creating a bad feeling between everyone—a perfect formula for a power struggle. You might end up arguing with everyone else but the picky eater. Insisting is a nagging, somewhat aggressive play and might just be about your own power and control mindset, not your child's. Check that.

Interactive Ways to Change Mealtime from Frantic to Fun

Make Healthy Choices Accessible

Furnish your toddler or school-aged child with some shelf space. Reserve a low shelf in the refrigerator for a variety of your toddler's favorite (nutritious) foods and drinks. Whenever she wants a snack, open the door and let her reach inside and choose one. This tactic also enables children to eat when they are hungry—an important step in acquiring a healthy attitude about food. This can also be an option for a non-refrigerated area of your home containing non-perishable foods. As crazy as this sounds, this is an additional a teaching opportunity. Your child will learn the first steps to becoming a self-functioning human. This small, self-governing step can empower children to problem-solve on their own. Children will become self-driven and a bit more independent though this tasking prospect. This is a great example of empowering your picky eater to make positive food choices.

Spread It . . . or Top It

Toddlers up to about six years old like smearing. Show them how to use a small disposable knife to spread cheese, peanut butter, or fruit jams onto crackers, toast or rice cakes. Toddlers are into toppings. Putting nutritious, familiar favorites on top of new and less-desirable foods is a way to broaden the finicky toddler's repertoire.

Don't worry about the mess. Children this age, depending on each individual, are still working on fine and gross motor skills. Remember to focus on the process, not the outcome. Baby wipes close by can quietly manage a mess if there is one. Encourage your child to grab a wet wipe and give them the opportunity to help with cleanup, yet another important task to teach.

Toddler Shots

If your youngster would rather drink than eat, don't despair; make a smoothie together. Milk and fruit, along with additions such as fresh juice, spinach, wheat germ, yogurt, honey and nut butters, can be the basis of very healthy meals. The kids can sip nutrition through a straw just as easily as chewing it. One note of caution: Avoid making smoothies with raw eggs, or you'll risk salmonella poisoning. Frozen fruit instead of ice can add more nutrition to a smoothie and keep things cold. Blueberries are a great way to turn green foods purple if your child will not touch anything resembling green foods. Just remember to talk about the green food in the drink when he accepts it. Don't be deceitful and lie about food.

Cuttin' Up

How much a child eats often depends on how you cut it. Cut sandwiches, pancakes, waffles and pizza into various shapes using cookie cutters. Think cocktail or tea party.

Dish It Out

Appearance is important. For something new and different, why not use your child's own toy plates for dishing out a snack? Kids enjoy the unexpected and fanciful when it comes to offering foods at the family table. But don't make a habit out of it.

Shop at Your Local Pet Supply Store

Yes, you read that correctly. This technique really worked for my kids. Young children are blessed with an active imagination and will imitate things they see, like cats, dogs and birds. If your child is an animal lover, she will definitely enjoy this imaginative role-playing technique. Simply take your picky eater to a local pet supply store and allow her to purchase a kitty or doggie bowl. Develop a casual agreement—if your child chooses to eat like a kitty or puppy, she has to choose from a reasonable menu or food types you both agree on together. Remember not to feed your child foods that she dislikes out of this vessel. Instead, meet the child halfway and have some fun with it. Teach your child about making compromises; don't make it a power struggle. And make sure your child understands that not every meal will be served in this vessel.

You could receive plenty of flak for this technique, but relax and let it happen. Your child is little; have fun! Presenting lunch in a kitty bowl and allowing your child to eat with his imagination can be a memory of a lifetime! You will enjoy interacting with your child's imagination, and your new technique will be sure to please.

This technique is easy because you can control what goes in the doggie or kitty dish. The deal is that she can only eat the agreed-upon foods from the pet bowls—stick to it. Begin with foods you know she will like. Build trust. Never give her something she will absolutely dislike in this dish. This dish will become an emblematic ring of trust. From there, the two of you can experiment. Never breech your child's trust by positioning foods and flavors or textures you know she will never love. Doing this could create a setback. It's not worth it. My kids never ate fish. I never forced it. Today, they are sushi eaters, but your child doesn't have to love everything you eat.

Make new food introductions an amusing, light, no-pressure effort. I went as far as painting kitty noses on the kids, but be careful not to allow this to become a daily event. Have your child pick a day of the week to eat out of his pet bowl. Just follow through and continue to discuss the negotiation—that he must eat all the food in the bowl. And remember to portion control and avoid a power struggle. Set the child up for a positive interaction with the new food rather than a failure; don't overload or place food in the dish that would be farfetched for any age to eat and enjoy. Do not confuse these fun-feeding activities with bribery.

Think Like a Chef—Presentation, Presentation, Presentation

Similar to allowing your child to partake in eating like a kitty cat, another great way to introduce your fussy toddler or seven-year-old to new food is to give her more control over serving herself. Offer her food in serving bowls and on platters family style, and allow her to choose what she wants. This gives her more freedom than having her food already placed on her plate, and she may be more likely to try something new.

Use the "pick two" closed-ended choice techniques here. When my children were three and four years old, they loved serving themselves when dinner was offered, especially when the giant serving platters with huge serving spoons were used for everyone's actual dinner plates. The girls would pile cucumber salad on their plates, looking at me every time they took a serving to make sure it was okay. I would say, "Go ahead, take as much as you want, but make sure you only take what you think you're going to eat." Subsequently, I could tell they felt empowered. They would sit back with strong postures, looking content with how grown-up they felt at choosing their own portions.

Neither of them touched the protein or any of the other vegetables. In fact, they did not even eat much of the cucumber salad, and they needed a few times to get a feel for their personal portions. I didn't try to convince them to eat, and those days they were comfortable eating only when prompted to do so.

Nothing was ever said about the pile of cucumbers or the fact that they weren't eating all of it. After a few family meals like this, the girls began to learn their capacity and take only what they could consume. Soon, without any pressure, they started to eat what they chose, and even tried some of the new foods I offered family style. The kids began to enjoy being in control, and they also appreciated knowing in advance what day of the week this would happen so they could emotionally prepare for it. Never surprise a picky eater. Ever.

No Surprise Parties

As adults, we don't like our supervisor or spouse coming to us with last-minute demands or unexpected duties. Surprises can place us in an uncomfortable position, such as your partner letting you know at the eleventh hour that unexpected guests are showing up at your home. Toddlers and younger kids feel the same way, so don't present them with a new food unexpectedly. Instead, plan for it. Plan new food celebrations one day a week— perhaps every Wednesday will be your family's "New Foods Wednesday." Children can emotionally plan for this day each week and not feel so out of control.

Use Sit Still Strategies

One reason why toddlers don't like to sit still at the family table is because their feet dangle. Try for yourself sitting on a stool while eating. You naturally begin to fidget and want to get up and move around. Children are likely to sit and eat longer at a child-size table and chair where their feet touch the floor. Make sure they are as comfortable as you and the rest of the family.

Turn Meals Upside Down

The distinctions between breakfast, lunch and dinner have little meaning to a child. If your youngster insists on eating pizza in the morning or fruit and cereal in the evening, go with it. Clearly this is better than not eating at all. This is not to say that you should become a short-order cook by filling lots of special requests, but why not let your toddler set the menu sometimes? Other family members will probably enjoy the novelty of waffles and protein-rich eggs for dinner. Allow everyone in the family to have a menu day. Of course, there should be reasonable expectations to this—that everyone agrees, within reason, to respect the food that is presented on that day and eat it.

Let Them Cook

Children are more likely to eat their own creations, so when the timing is appropriate, let your child help prepare the food. Use cookie cutters to create edible designs out of foods like cheese, bread, thin meat slices, or cooked lasagna noodles. Give your pint-size assistant such jobs as dumping in ingredients, stirring, tearing and washing lettuce, scrubbing potatoes, or mixing items together. Put pancake batter in a squeeze bottle and let your child supervise as you squeeze the batter onto the hot griddle in fun shapes like hearts, numbers, letters or even words.

Share It

If your child is going through a picky-eater stage, invite a friend over who is the same age or slightly older and you know "likes to eat." Your child will catch on. Group feedings are great because it allows the other kids to set the example.

Become a Chef; Play Restaurant

A common complaint among parents is their concern that their child won't eat vegetables; yet, despite the parents' distress, the child keeps growing. How does this happen? Don't worry. Vegetables require some creative marketing, and eventually kids will develop a taste for them. Play with your child, and ask them to engage in a restaurant simulation and prepare the family menu together. When other family members arrive home, take their order, but remember to use closed-ended choices when planning the menu, and set an example of a balanced meal containing proteins, grains and vegetables. Choose similar flavors to foods they already enjoy. Think outside the box. Cook from scratch on these days. And don't give up on the first try.

Just Chill

Foods that are colder temperatures won't have as much of an impact on tiny tongues.[9] Some kids' taste receptors can be intensified at least ten times more than adults, especially bitter taste receptors. If you suspect this is what's happening with your child, serve foods a bit colder than usual.

This is how I introduced green peas to my children. They snacked on frozen peas because it was a novelty— and the cold food was a subtle introduction to the pungent green flavors. As my children became accustomed to the green flavor, I started to thaw them to a very cold temperature. At that point, I suggested how fun it was to hear the peas pop in our mouths when we chewed them. As time grew, their green repertoire grew.

Peas are a great start into the world of green foods because they are naturally sweet. Today, I think fresh peas are my children's favorite vegetable. It's possible that they associate the food with fun times. If it is, I'm glad they emotionally associate with a green pea rather than an empty calorie food.

Grow a Garden with Your Child

Gardening is a wonderful opportunity for kids to witness the full cycle of vegetables from seed to harvest. Let your child help care for the plants, harvest the ripe vegetables, and wash and prepare them. He will become more interested in eating what he has helped nurture and grow.

Grate Vegetables into Favorite Foods

Add grated vegetables to rice, cottage cheese, cream cheese, guacamole, or even macaroni and cheese for an extra nutritional

---

9   Monell Chemical Senses Center, "Children's Taste Sensitivity And Food Choices Influenced By Taste Gene," *ScienceDaily*, 18 February 2005.

punch. Zucchini pancakes and carrot muffins are a big hit, too. Most kids love salads; thinly-cut lettuces and grated solid veggies make salads fun for little ones. Allow children to prepare their own dressing. Give them a whisk to mix up a simple sweet-and-salty umami vinaigrette. The salad dressing that they help create will not only make them curious regarding the flavor, but also make them proud to present the recipe to the rest of the family. Usually, salad dressings made with apple cider or rice vinegars appeal to a toddler's sensitivity to bitter flavors because they are a bit milder. And balsamic vinegars are sweet. Keep your salad dressings cold for kids with sensitive palates.

If your child assists you in the kitchen, make sure she works safe. Place a damp towel on the child's work surface under the bowl or under a cutting board so there is a non-slip surface for the child to work on. This also makes for easy clean up; lift the cutting board or bowl and there is a wet towel to clean with. I love little time-saving tips in the kitchen. We all need them.

Don't Overdo It

Boiling vegetables reduces the nutrients and makes food unappealing. If you must boil, only cook part of the way, and have a bowl of ice water in the sink waiting. With a slotted spoon, remove the vegetable from the boiling water and place it into the cold ice bath. This is called "shocking" the vegetable. It will cool the cooking process quickly and lock in nutrients. You will notice vibrant color immediately. When you are ready to serve, gently reheat and serve at room temperature or chilled.

Try steaming your greens, or stir-fry. Steaming or stir-frying vegetables helps bring out delicious flavor—stir-frying brings out natural sugars in foods. The browning of the food is actually the natural sugar content caramelizing with the addition of heat, thus making foods sweeter than if they were served raw. Basil is a good starter herb to introduce to children because it's sweet and smells wonderfully fragrant. Basil pesto colors scrambled eggs really green, which makes it fun and healthy. I always try to avoid using food coloring or anything artificial not found in nature. Slipping basil pesto into the pan at the last minute will provide enough heat time to explode the flavor without killing the nutrients or making the food look unappealing. Small little food processors can whip up a green basil pesto in no time and with little mess. Basil pesto can be stored in the fridge for additions to meals later in the week when time counts; or you can place leftover pesto in ice cube trays and freeze for later use. Read Dr. Seuss's *Green Eggs and Ham* before introducing pesto to toddlers; they will really enjoy it!

Make Veggie Art

Some picky eaters just need this little extra fun. Create colorful faces with sliced olives as eyes, tomato ears, mushroom noses, bell-pepper mustaches, and any other playful features you can think of. (Remember, as a child, how you loved to put olives on the tip of each finger?) Zucchini pancakes make terrific faces to which you can add pea eyes, a carrot nose, and cheese hair.

Lies and Camouflages

Again, I mention this subject because being dishonest can require serious damage control later. There are all kinds of variations on the old standby, "cheese in the forest" (cheese melted on steamed broccoli florets), or you can enjoy veggies topped with peanut sauce—a delicious Asian cultural specialty. These camouflages are fine. Explain to your child what is being presented. Some parents wait until after the child tastes before they present the menu descriptions; however, at no point will I suggest that you hide or lie about the foods you serve your kids. Presenting undesirable types of foods in different formats might make a difference (e.g., serve cheeses melted instead of cold or sauces made with milk instead of water or juices). A food pairing can make a difference with foods that are not necessarily enjoyed alone. However, when certain foods are paired up, the umami sense can kick in and create a completely different taste on your tongue. This is something food scientists have been studying for years. See more on umami in Chapter Nine: The Advanced Battle.

The Family Meal

Of course, it won't be possible to sit together as a family for every meal, but make an effort to eat together for at least one meal a day. Toddlers and preschoolers learn by imitating, and the best way to develop healthy eating habits is from watching you. If you are eating oodles of vegetables and healthy foods, this will seem normal and familiar to your child, and he is more likely to eat them also. Toddlers and young children are copycats! This can also be a wonderful time to be together as a family and give your child the attention she craves. If you have successfully eliminated the pressure and nagging with regard to food, eating together can actually be a wonderful experience.

Keep in mind that toddlers and preschoolers have short attention spans and they may not be willing or able to sit for a prolonged period of time; however, continue to encourage her to sit with the family, even if she says she isn't hungry, and don't pressure her to eat. This is a good time to have a conversation, ask questions about her day, and give her an opportunity to eat and relax with you in a calm and loving environment, especially older children. Ask open-ended questions to stimulate conversation.

Very young children are distracted easily; if they are left alone to eat at the table, they can lose focus and end up leaving the table or just playing with their food. When the family sits together, you can focus on each other and your meal.

Suggestions to promote conversation:

What was the best thing that happened to you today?
What was the best of the best that happened to you today?
What was the hardest rule to follow today?
Who made you smile today?
What made your teacher smile today?
What made your teacher frown today?
What was the worst thing that happened to you today?
Who did you sit with at lunch today?
Was anyone absent from your class today?
What kind of person were you today?

Did you do anything creative today?

If you could change anything about today, what would it be?

Instead of beginning a conversation with "How was your day today," stimulate conversation and create a positive, bonding, family mealtime experience for everyone, including you.

Toddler Manners

Younger toddlers like to explore new foods by touching them, inspecting them and, in some cases, squishing them before depositing anything in their little mouths. Let them. This is an important part of the process for this age group. They should outgrow this within a year or two.

Remember, new foods are foreign to little people, who are used to eating everything mashed up. Let them squish their banana and crumble their cubes of cheese. As long as they are allowed to touch and experience the new foods, the chances are better they will be less anxious to try them.

Preschoolers sometimes need to use their fingers to push their food onto their forks. They are still acquiring motor skill coordination at this age, and their little hands and fingers make it difficult for them to use their cutlery properly. Let them explore their food with their hands as well, as long as they are not throwing food on the floor, at family members, or smashing it onto the table and making a complete mess.

It is important for even very young children to learn to say "please" and "thank you" and be polite when they are sitting and eating jointly with you or with a group. This is an excellent opportunity to help them learn these fundamental social skills. Of course, there will still be tantrums and crying and attempted negotiations around the food, but as long as you stay calm and don't get caught up in the course of events surrounding these tantrums, you can just remind them that their behavior isn't acceptable at the table. Do not give any further attention to it unless they are being so disruptive that they need to be removed from the table. If this is the case, just apply a natural consequence.

Keep in mind: If you are off the scheduled feeding time

or the day went later than expected and your child missed a naptime, these things can all influence a child to act out during mealtime. In this case it really is not the child's fault. Try to be fair when removing them from the table. Maybe it's an early bath and bedtime she needs instead of a time-out. Every situation will be different, and you should take everything into account before drawing conclusions on why your child is not eating at a schedule mealtime.

When They Are Hungry, They Will Eat

All children will eat and drink when they are hungry. Apply closed-ended choices, be patient and realistic, think about the effectiveness of timing, and remember the size of their little bellies. Avoid offering new foods to a fatigued picky eater and your life will be less taxing. Be good to yourself and remember that your role is important and to remain patient.

Chapter Nine

THE ADVANCED BATTLE | ELICITING SCIENCE

For those parents who are interested in accepting a scientific gastronomic approach to picky eating and would like to begin adding a rare, all-natural flavor sensation to foods, here is some information on how. But first, a little of the science behind flavor.

Umami /oo-mommy/ *noun*: A taste sensation that is savory.

We all have the four primary tastes: sweetness, sourness, bitterness and saltiness.[10] There is also a fifth taste—not on our tongues but within certain foods. It's referred to as umami.

There are plenty of foods in which umami occur naturally, including meat, fish, vegetables and dairy. Some kids might enjoy these experiences, but some kids might not, so experiment with typical food pairings to see what works for your child.

When humans eat, they use all their senses to form judgments

---

10   Menche N. (ed.) Biologie Anatomie Physiologie. Munich: Urban & Fischer/ Elsevier; 2012. Pschyrembel W. Klinisches Wörterbuch. Berlin: De Gruyter; 2014. Schmidt R, Lang F, Heckmann M. Physiologie des Menschen: mit Pathophysiologie. Heidelberg: Springer; 2011.

about foods, but taste is the most significant out of your five human senses. Enhancing the sense of taste by adding umami-flavored ingredients can actually change the flavor sensation on our tongue.

Chances are that you are already a big fan of umami but don't know it yet. Umami is helpful in creating flavor combinations that make your tongue and your brain happy, so with a little bit of knowledge about which foods naturally contain the fifth taste, you can get the same hard-to-put-your-finger-on sensation. Most food pairings engage the sweet and salty portions of the tongue.

In prehistoric history, the resilient link bonding taste with emotion is really about human evolution. Taste has always been a survival sense. Taste helped us identify the food we were consuming. A bitter or sour taste indicated poisonous or inedible plant-based material. Taste also helped us identify decomposing, protein-rich food. Sweet and salty tastes are attractive and often a sign our food is rich in nutrients. The umami taste, which is somewhat similar to the taste of a meat broth, is usually caused by glutamic acid or aspartic acid.[11] These two amino acids are part of many different proteins found in food and also in some plants. Ripe tomatoes, meat, and Parmesan cheese all contain extraordinary allocations of glutamic acid. Asparagus contains aspartic acid.

Have you ever enjoyed sweet and salty flavors mixed together, such as salty pretzels dipped into compote or plunged into melted chocolate? Have you tried fresh pears and strong-smelling cheese combinations? These types of food pairings can create the sensation of umami.

Try this adult experiment: Choose a mediocre-tasting white zinfandel and take a sip. Savor the flavor. Next, eat an acidic green olive (one you would place into a martini.) Now, take another taste of the wine. You will notice that the mediocre white zinfandel suddenly tastes miraculous. This change in taste is actually an umami experience.

This remarkable taste sensation often happens with foods that are naturally rich in glutamates (see the list below). Glutamate is found in our brain and is responsible for normal brain functions like cognitive development, memory and learning. It is also

---

11   Shizuko Yamaguchi, and Kumiko Ninomiya, "What is umami?" *Food Reviews International* 14, no.2–3 (1998).

responsible for cellular survival. It is considered to be the major moderator of excitatory signals in our central nervous system. In other words, these foods make us happy, happy, and happy!

Keep in mind that your children have thousands of additional taste buds, so flavor sensations can be extremely overwhelming. Especially bitter flavors.

I love to introduce umami to picky eaters' parents because it creates a pleasant savory taste and blends well with other flavors. Umami expands and rounds out flavors. Most people cannot recognize umami flavors, so your child will never know you have created a delicious flavor using a dash of fish sauce or dried fish flakes or a sprinkling of mushroom powder or tomato paste. I'm not advocating lying about food; however, if your child is squeamish about using such condiments, just place more emphasis on the other flavor profiles in the dish. If he is old enough to understand, explain umami and anchor a bit of science education to your mealtimes.

Not all kids will love the protein-rich meats and seafood high in umami, so I have listed several foods high in glutamate that picky eaters are more likely to enjoy.

Umami Home Pantry

The following is a list of the most umami-friendly ingredients that can be used in almost any dish to ramp up flavors.

Parmesan Cheese

Sprinkle grated cheeses into scrambled eggs, omelets, soups, sauces, stews, and vegetable or starchy side dishes. And don't throw away that rock-hard cheese rind that you cannot grate. Toss it into soups, sauces and stews as they simmer, and let it release its flavor. When cheesemongers ripen cheese, it loses water, thus becoming harder and saltier. As a result, cheese flavor becomes stronger and more complex. In addition, you taste a stronger umami; aging causes protein in cheese to break down into amino acids, further increasing the content of glutamate, one of the luxurious umami sources.

Fish Sauce

Used sparingly, there's less aroma, and the umami boost is spectacular. If you like Thai food, notably pad Thai and *tom yum gai* (Thai chicken soup), the umami blast from fish sauce is a major reason why you find it so delicious. Try a splash or two in soups, marinades, salad dressings, pasta dishes and casseroles. The Thai variety is called *nam pla*; the Vietnamese variety is *nuoc mam* (and some say it is an enhanced version). I have tested these sauces with my students over the years at my culinary school, and, surprisingly, many gulped up foods containing *dashi* or fish sauces. It's almost magic.

Shiitake Mushrooms

Soak dry mushrooms in warm water for about 20 minutes to reconstitute, then chop and add to soups and sauces. Filter the soaking liquid right into the pan or save for adding to soups and stews or deglazing a pan; it's loaded with umami taste.

Pulverize dried shiitake mushrooms in a blender and sprinkle the resulting powder on steamed vegetables, or coat a roast with it before popping it in the oven. You can also search online and purchase shiitake mushroom substrates seeded with mushroom spores. Together you and your child can grow your own fascinating fungi. I often use mushroom powder and sprinkle it like I would with salt and pepper. Definitely a chef's secret weapon.

Soy Sauce

Insist on naturally-brewed soy sauce. Use a dollop in stews, meatloaf, hamburgers, braised vegetables, marinades, salad dressings and dipping sauces. Just a touch adds an umami lift; a little more adds a pleasant Asian flavor to your meals. Be sure to adjust your salt in recipes accordingly. Some soy sauces render a salty flavor.

Worcestershire Sauce

This ubiquitous condiment derives most of its umami from the glutamate-rich anchovies in its customary recipe. Use it the same ways as soy sauce.

Canned Tomatoes

Specifically, top-quality Italian canned tomatoes. Aside from their use in tomato sauce, canned tomatoes add an umami kick to soups and sides that are otherwise dull. Choose whole, crushed or sauce, depending on the texture you want in the finished dish. Great to use in homemade ketchup with your child, the umami affluence in cherry tomatoes is high. After swallowing a high-glutamate ingredient, you will still feel your mouth watering. Umami affects salivation.

Meats

Red meats tend to be higher in umami than others. Aging, curing, and drying meats generally intensifies the umami taste. Some examples include prosciutto and ham; however, umami can also be found in chicken and pork. Dry-cured ham is one of the most umami-rich ingredients you can find. You may feel a strong aftertaste of umami. Some manufactures use an ingredient for curing ham called inosinate, which is rich in umami. If you are avoiding anything processed, then cured meats are not going to be your thing. There are also naturally occurring enzymes that are present during the long period of maturing dry-cured meats. You can also look for a company that processes naturally. Other enzymes break down protein into amino acids. Glutamate is a naturally occurring amino acid that actually increases with age.

Fish

Small fish, such as anchovies and sardines, are high in umami, as are red-fleshed fish such as tuna and cod. Again, processing seems to intensify the flavor. Dried and fermented fish products have excessive levels of umami.

Other Seafood

Scallops, clams, shrimp, squid, oysters and other foods of the sea tend to be high in umami. Oyster sauce is a common way of harnessing this flavor; this is why stir-fries are often popular with kids. Oyster sauce is a sweet and savory sauce with a deep, earthy flavor provided by oyster juices that have been cooked down and caramelized. Caramelization is the browning of naturally occurring sugars in an ingredient; cooking extensively will result in a sweet, nutty flavor and brown color.

Seaweed and Kelp

From dashi broth to the *nori* seaweed your sushi is wrapped in, these options are attractive to a small child's palette. I've noticed that some kids won't eat seafood but love to munch on nori products. These products can usually be found in the specialty foods isle at your local supermarket or ordered online. Dashi is a simple and savory Japanese stock, usually made from *kombu* (kelp), *katsuobushi* (dried bonito flakes, i.e., dried, fermented, and smoked skipjack tuna shaved into paper-thin flakes), and sometimes shiitake mushrooms, and cared for as reverently as a round of Parmesan cheese in Parma, Italy. This simple yet umami-rich taste is indispensable to Japanese cuisine.

Vegetables

Some umami-rich vegetables include tomatoes, carrots, capers (I call them umami bombs), Chinese cabbage, sweet potatoes, potatoes, truffles, soybeans and shiitake mushrooms.

Other Products

In addition to the foods already listed, chicken, eggs and green tea provide umami flavors. You can cook in green tea by adding the liquid to soups, casseroles and sauces. Check for caffeine levels prior.

You are likely thinking your child would *never* eat any of these umami items. I am not advocating that you solely rely on these ingredients but rather that you integrate them into your cooking when you can and experience the metamorphosis of taste for yourself. No matter what the studies reveal, the truth is that we are all living in a world of processed and high-calorie food choices; today, more than ever, it is important that we pay closer attention to what our children are eating and when. Umami can assist us in preparing home-cooked meals booming with flavor.

Chapter Ten

NEW FOODS AND CHILDREN WITH SPECIAL NEEDS

For the first time in the history, obesity and being overweight are increasingly prevalent in the general pediatric population. According to the American Association of Pediatrics, evidence suggests that children with special needs, especially children with autism spectrum disorder (ASD), may be at an even higher elevated risk for unhealthy weight gain, with differences present as early as ages two to five. To make matters worse, these results clearly indicated that the prevalence of unhealthy weight is significantly greater among special needs children, compared with the general population.

A study published in 2008 by the US Library of Medicine's National Institution on Health listed childhood obesity as a problem affecting nearly one-third of US children. The dominance of this condition has increased at least fourfold since the 1970s.

Obesity in kids with special needs and ASD may be

particularly problematic for an assortment of reasons.[12] First, primary symptoms may be naturally related to weight problems; for instance, these children may lack social motivation to participate in family meals or in systematized physical activities with other children, and parents may be more likely to use food as a reward for children with special needs due to lack of social motivation. The severity or type of a child's symptoms may also affect his ability to participate in physical activities that mitigate weight gain.

Still, it is unclear whether risk factors for obesity in special needs children or kids with ASD are the same or different from risk factors for children generally.

Good nutrition and special needs children rarely go hand in hand easily. Often, parents who are responsible for mealtimes within a special needs family concentrate on what the neuro-typical world does not. Special needs parents live with higher instances of restricted eating and, especially in ASD children, a repetitive pattern of behavior associated with food. ASD parents are also faced with a higher intake of low-nutrition, energy-dense foods. Parents usually give in and pick their battles elsewhere. Can't say that I blame them. I've done it myself.

Ready, Set . . . Go

Before making any changes, think back on what your child repetitively eats. Maybe it's a fast food item—something introduced into his diet before you realized it was time for a change. Identify that item. Begin to build other foods to look like it in shape as well as color. Example: Making homemade organic baked chicken tenderloins shorter and breaded in gluten free bread crumbs to look like the fast food chicken nuggets you are trying to wean him off. Take all the time you need. Make sure this process is moving at the speed your child is absorbing the solution. Take each step a day at a time or once a week on the same day each week.

---

12   Cynthia L. Ogden, PhD; Margaret D. Carrll, MSPH; Lester R. Curtin, PhD; et al, "Prevalence of Overweight and Obesity in the United States, 1999-2004," *JAMA* 295, no. 13 (2006):1549-1555.

Always prepare your child, and *never* lie or be deceitful or sneaky about food. Not to make parenting more stressful, but it all stops here, with us: the parents. It is our responsibility to teach our children to eat safely, using clean ingredients, and to keep our children healthy emotionally as well as physically. As if our jobs are not hard enough, we add a picky or selective eater to our daunting, ever-growing lineup of duties. Some days it seems as though we will never score a few points in our favor, let alone win the food fight.

For many parents, loading healthy nutrition into your picky or selective eater's diet will always be a mealtime battle. Because special needs kids all have a unique lifestyle, we all need to run our own battery of food testing. Sensory issues can make introducing new and nutritious foods extremely hard for parents. Children who like repetition and routines each day provide another interesting challenge. Oral sensitivity issues can also make this difficult situation worse.

Whether you are a new parent or a seasoned special needs parent and you need to make a nutritional change, please ask your doctor before starting a new food regimen. Most families find going gluten and casein free really helps. Lose fast food as quickly as you can. Try to stay dye-free and offer organic, minimally-processed food replacements. Make this part of the whole family's repertoire. Read labels. Cook at home every chance you have. Avoid highly processed foods at all costs.

It is common for special needs kids to have allergies. Usually, if a child rejects a certain food, the body is speaking. Your child's body will naturally reject certain foods for a myriad of reasons. Again, pay close attention to those cues. Whatever is causing these reactions should stay off the menu forever. Your child's body will naturally attack a food it identifies as harmful, causing symptoms such as nausea, stomach pain, intestinal integrity, shortness of breath, hives. With food intolerance, the digestive system alone rejects the food, finding it difficult to digest properly. Follow the food cues. If struggling to gain leverage in new food acceptance, try my ten-step process below.

Ten Steps to Introducing New Foods

- Begin a food journal. Inside the food journal, build a list containing two columns. In the first column, list the foods that your child enjoys eating. Use the other column to list a healthier alternative for each food listed in the first column. Keep another list recording the dates you offer the foods.

- Remember, children are always watching and listening, even if you think they are not. Your family's words and actions can make or break just about anything. Spread the message among family members regarding your new food fight strategy.

- Eat the desired new food while sitting next to your child, and comment on how delicious the food tastes while the child is observing you eating and enjoying the new food. Remember—if you are not eating it, don't expect your child to.

- Peer Pressure. Have a friend of the child, or a highly reinforcing person, eat the food next to the child and make positive comments. Again, make sure your child is actually paying close attention.

- During therapy, downtime, or homework hour, place a photo of the desired food into the mix of whatever the child is working on. Make the food photo a tactile flashcard, not a photo from your phone. Prepare one photo flashcard for each new food. Use one at a time or a few, depending on your child's tolerance. Play a flashcard game. Look at the food picture and talk about the new food. Mention the food's name, what it tastes like, how delicious it is, where it comes from, and who else eats it.

- When you have cycled through a few flashcard activities, add the actual food to the flashcard lineup. Just touch it, look at it, feel it, and discuss how delicious it tastes. Discuss the ways people cook and eat the new food. Describe and identify textures.

- Once you have cycled through the flashcard game enough times and the child has actually seen the new food, now is the time to place a small amount of the new food on a plate at the next mealtime. Place the new food on a separate plate close to the child's dinner plate during mealtimes. Point to the new food and discuss it. Talk about how delicious it is and allow the child to see you eat it and enjoy it. Do not make the child touch or eat the food at this time.

- Place a small amount of the new food on the child's plate with his regular meal. Make sure this is a not a surprise, and create a no-pressure zone. Tell the child before you put the new food on the plate, using the name of the food, and tell the child he does not have to eat the new food, but he needs to tolerate the food sitting on his plate during the course of the mealtime.

- Place the same food item on the child's plate and, during mealtimes, tell the child he needs to touch the food. Tell the child he does not have to eat the food; the food only needs to be touched with a finger once during the mealtime.

- Continue the process until the food is tasted. Remain patient. The process of adding a new repertoire of foods won't happen overnight, but it will happen.

- By the end of a four to eight month period, you might have them eating many foods from the healthy food column you designed, including organic, grass-fed, nitrate-free hamburger meats; new, healthier variations of chicken; or fresh fish nuggets, and lots of real fruits and vegetables in their natural form. Each child is different. Be patient. In the long run, you and your family will find peace of mind, free from the additional health issues associated with eating highly-processed foods.

Chapter Eleven

NEW BEGINNINGS | A HEALTHIER LIFESTYLE

L et's stop for a moment and consider what the phrase "good eater" mean to you. Does it mean that your child eats what is given to him and cleans his plate without protest? Does it mean that you can take your child to a cultural smorgasbord and have him load up on curry, spicy burritos and pad Thai? Does it mean that the child will always at least try anything he is served?

Being a decent eater means different things to different parents, but the common denominator is that we all want our children to be healthy, both physically and mentally. We worry that they are not getting enough nutrition, and that they are subject to developing complications with food and could someday become anorexic, bulimic or overweight.

I hope I've demonstrated to you that it is possible for your child to have a positive, healthy relationship with food and eating. All it takes is a new perspective. Give up your old concepts about feeding, and emerge with a new blueprint. Swear off fast food restaurants, begin reading labels, educate yourself on what is actually going into your family's bodies, and make mealtimes a positive, significant time of the day for the whole family. Most of all, do not engage in a battle.

Enrich Childhood Memories

Food is associated with culture, tradition and special occasions. Many of us remember foods our grandparents prepared when we visited, or special feasts enjoyed when company arrived, or foods prepared during celebrations. When we let go of the melee around food and embrace how it nourishes us not only physically but also spiritually, our kids will do the same. Let's face it: Food is one of life's greatest pleasures.

Build Vocabulary Around Snack and Mealtimes

Rich conversations happen at mealtimes. When we introduce new and exciting foods, we can also talk about what we're eating and often how it's presented or the geography behind it as well as the science. We can talk to our kids about where the food came from or how it was grown and how it has evolved through ancient cultures. Present new vocabulary—words like *succulent*, *poach*, *braise*, and *grill*, *palate*, *aroma* and *puree* and more. Mealtime is often the only time a family can gather and connect. It's a period when we share the highlights of our day and check in with one another. A child's vocabulary expands when we make a habit of engaging him in conversation. This intimate moment additionally presents an opportunity to offer words of praise, support and encouragement.

Begin transitioning the whole family into safer and healthier nutrition choices. Switching to an advantageous diet can be challenging with a picky eater, so the sooner you introduce this concept to fledgling children the better. As parents and caregivers, it is up to us to teach the subsequent generation to make improved choices, and healthy eating is much easier to implement preemptively than to modify later.

We live in a society today where our families are continuously under the attack of marketing and advertisements to entice children and ourselves to make poor nutrition decisions. Television, magazines, supermarkets, commercials, billboard and internet ads all offer us options that are detrimental to our health and our family's health.

Children over the age of two should limit their intake of saturated fats, sugars and foods high in sodium.[13] Limit fast or processed foods, which are usually high in fats, sugars, sodium, fillers, and may contain nutritionally inferior ingredients.

Many grocery stores are stocked with food high in artificial preservatives to keep foods on the shelves longer and food containing artificial coloring to make foods look more attractive or more food-like. All of these items listed may have adverse effects on your family health. Fast food restaurants almost always serve foods high in saturated fat, sugar and sodium. Serving sizes should always questioned in a fast food restaurant. Single-order containers such as a potato fries container are overfilled or contain enough for two servings, and we never read the fine print or a nutrition label. The larger servings are attractive, instantaneously convincing the purchasers they are achieving value when they are really only receiving additional calories from nutritionally vacant foods. Preparing and eating whole foods from home will always be a healthier option.

Help! What to do if . . .

Your child says he isn't hungry

So, your family has finally made a change in eating style and you are taking control, supplying healthy choices and removing fast food from mealtimes. Now your child suggests he is not hungry when it's a scheduled mealtime because he really doesn't want to eat the new foods.

Encourage your child to come and sit at the table anyway so you can visit with him. Explain to your child that dinner is a time for the family to be together. When the child comes to the table, make sure you follow the rules: Offer the child some food, and then don't say another word about it. If the child hops up after ten minutes and says he is full, even if he hasn't eaten a bite, let him go. However, don't feed the child again until the

13 American Academy of Pediatrics Committee on Nutrition, "Prevention of pediatric overweight and obesity." *Pediatrics* 112, no. 2 (August 2003): 424-430.

next scheduled snack, and remind him why he's hungry when he asks for a bedtime snack.

Again, it is really a case-by-case basis. What did the child eat during the day? When was the last mealtime? Is the child drinking juice or milk all day? Is he participating in sports? How old is he? These are all questions that need to be answered before a course of action can be decided.

Your child refuses to sit still at the table

In terms of squirming and not sitting up straight, if it isn't hurting anyone and the chair isn't in danger of being broken by being pushed back on two legs, ignore it. Young children have a lot of excess energy, and it can be difficult for them to sit still. If you find that she is obviously just not hungry anymore and can't seem to contain her energy, you can suggest that it might be time for her to get up and go play. However, make sure that she realizes that she won't eat again until her next snack. You don't want her hopping up and down from the table every three minutes, or it turns into a game. She sits and eats for the time allotted for her level of attentiveness. As suggested earlier, make sure that your child's little feet are not dangling. Dangling feet can give the child an unusual sense of needing movement. If she's new to the toddler stage, chances are she will be a complete wanderer until three years of age and she will only sit for a short amount time. You can also incorporate a timer into this scenario and teach the child she must sit at the table for a specific period of time. Be engaging. Include her in conversations. Nothing worse than being a kid sitting at the table after the meal has been eaten listening to adult-talk. Remember—adult time and child time are two entirely different times.

Your child wants something other than what's being served

This can be very heart wrenching, but you need to stick to your convictions for your child's sake. If the meal you are serving is not something your toddler or preschooler wants to eat, or you are weaning a school-aged child off fast or processed foods, tell him that this is the meal you made for the family, everyone in the family is expected to eat it, and no other meals will be made just for him. However, if he would like to participate in what meals should be served, make a family activity and design a weekly menu together.

Describe the features and benefits of eating better and how everything can improve, including skills in any sport the child might be participating in. Healthful nourishment can be part of a plan to gain energy and focus, play harder, increase strength and so on. This will be especially difficult if the child is used to having a grilled cheese sandwich every night or going to the drive-through. After the child's initial anger and frustration and, yes, even fear, he will realize that this is the way it's going to be. Don't give in—that just confuses your child even more, and he will think that, if he cries or screams loud enough, eventually you will cave.

Keep in mind that it's a good idea to always serve something that your child likes along with the rest of the meal, even if it's only bread and butter. At least then he will feel that he has an option if he can't bring himself to try whatever you've made that night. Don't worry. The more secure the child feels and the less he believes that eating is something he has to do to make you happy, the more likely he is to try new foods. Following through is the key. Doing this a few times will put the short-order cook out of service! Save yourself, and help your child learn lifelong healthy habits.

You have tried everything and cannot get your child to eat anything new

It is time to deploy the advanced battle techniques. See my ten-step process in Chapter Ten.

Chapter Twelve

BATTLE BREAKFAST

For growing little bodies, breakfast often includes fruit or vegetables, a carbohydrate like cereal or rice, protein, sometimes dairy, and a beverage. The Journal of the American College of Nutrition has referred to breakfast as the most important meal of the day; studies find that people who skip breakfast are more likely to have problems with concentration, metabolism and weight management. Adults are often guilty of skipping breakfast, with many of us preferring to grab a cup of coffee and go. However, if we let our kids follow our bad habits, we're depriving them of the opportunity to get their day off to a healthy start.

Breakfast, if you take the time to serve it, could actually be one of the only meals your toddler or preschooler eats without a fuss. His little tummy is empty when he wakes up, so he's more willing to eat. Many of the common breakfast foods are typically foods that young children like, such as fruit, yogurt, toast and cereal.

How your family handles the first meal of the day will depend on many factors: the age of your child, whether you work or stay at home with the kids, and your child's particular hunger patterns and morning stress levels.

In keeping with the whole no-pressure approach, I'm not suggesting that you force your preschooler to choke down a big bowl of oatmeal before he hits the playground, but rather that you use some of the skills already outlined to make breakfast a painless and enjoyable experience for your child, and for you too!

Breakfast Myths

A healthy breakfast should be hot or cooked

Not necessarily. In fact, many parents are just too busy to cook for their kids on weekday mornings: leftovers, fruit, yogurt, even cheese and crackers are all perfectly acceptable and nutritious. If your child likes hot food for breakfast and you're in a hurry, cooking rolled oats can be fast and still keep you away from crazy additives found in those little instant pouches. I can whip out a warm oatmeal breakfast in less than five minutes with oats. Oatmeal with milk is a good choice, as well as waffles you can place in a toaster or toaster oven (avoid toaster pastries, which are loaded with sugar). I would make a batch of homemade waffles and pancakes on the weekends and freeze them for midweek—so simple to pop into the toaster when you are on the go. Top with a bit of nut butter and fresh fruit, and you have a great beginning to the day. Don't overlook eggs. Eggs can be fried or scrambled fairly quickly. Whatever you decide, just make sure not to undercook them; there's nothing worse than runny, slimy egg if you are a picky eater.

I don't recommend the precooked bacon and sausage products. But I do recommend you precook bacon and make sausage patties on the weekends for a quick midweek heat up. You can also assemble wholesome breakfast burritos and freeze those too. At least you will know what is inside, and they will not be full of artificial ingredients.

Store-bought premade bacon, sausages, breakfast sandwiches, and breakfast burritos will contain high sodium content as well as loads of shelf stabilizers and preservatives. A few great companies prepare nitrate-free products, which is another reason to read labels thoroughly. Search for the best products possible for your family and make them your go-to options. I know how much work it is to get the kids up, washed, dressed, fed and out the door in the morning. If you need to use a premade product occasionally, that is okay—we do the best we can with the amount of time we have. Make small modifications, a little at a time. And don't be too hard on yourself if you have a setback in food choices. You already have a big job taking care of the family. Take one day at a time.

Planning is everything. On the weekends, take some time to plan a meal-prep session. Cook up several extra waffles or pancakes and freeze them individually, and then pop them into airtight storage. Assemble toasted English muffins with cooked eggs and cheese, wrap them up and freeze them, pull them out midweek to thaw in the fridge the night before, and boom—you have fast food that is *real* food, wholesome without the fast food mystery meats and preservatives. Hot breakfast foods can be wrapped in foil to keep the heat in on busy days, and the kids can eat it in the car with a 100 percent fruit juice box in hand.

Breakfast must contain breakfast foods

Some of us are under the impression that breakfast always consists of hot or cold cereal, fruit, toast, bacon or eggs. Not true! In fact, in most Asian countries, breakfast is almost identical to dinner and lunch, with common choices being rice with vegetables or meat, as well as soups and curries.

Serve dinner for breakfast! I do. There's absolutely nothing wrong with your four-year-old eating last night's spaghetti and a glass of milk for breakfast. After all, homemade pizza, for instance, covers protein, grains and dairy products. Serve sliced apple or pear on the side and your child has a perfectly balanced meal that tastes great. Other selections to consider include a grilled cheese sandwich, leftover pasta, or a warm bowl of your child's beloved soup.

Traditional Breakfast Choices

Cold Cereals

When selecting a cold cereal, avoid choosing one that lists sugar as a main ingredient.

Check the nutritional information on all boxes of cereal; odds are that you'll find one you and your kids can agree on. Some cereals that contain very high daily-recommended vitamin and mineral amounts are lavish and unnecessary. No need to blow your food budget on high-end cereals. Your kids are going to be eating throughout the day and will have ample opportunity to load up on the calcium, fiber and iron they need; these nutrients certainly don't need to come from one bowl of cereal. If you must serve dry cereal, search the healthy isle of your grocery store and read labels. Don't allow marketers to entertain you or your child. If you are shopping and your child is with you, avoid visiting the cereal aisle. You will thank me later!

Hot Cereals

Oatmeal is a common favorite, and you can add raisins, cinnamon, brown sugar, berries, chopped almonds, walnuts, sunflower seeds and anything else you can think of. If your child doesn't like oatmeal, try polenta, hot rice, or wheat cereal. They are easy to make in the microwave or on the stovetop. Don't depend on instants.

Fruit

Sliced apple, pear, banana, orange, pineapple and melon look attractive on a plate, and when berries are in season, most kids will eat them by the handful. Whatever you have on hand is great, and if you can offer a couple of choices, even better. If your child is not in the mood for sliced fruit, applesauce or fresh fruit, cooked compotes can be an additional option, but try to avoid added sugar.

Grains

Toast is a common favorite in the morning. Frozen waffles are popular if you cannot prepare them from scratch ahead of time and freeze them. Pancakes, bagels and croissants are a hit with kids and high in carbohydrates to fuel the busy morning ahead. Younger kids really like mini-bagels, which are more appropriate in size for their little bellies. Cream cheese is a good dairy protein to spread; mild goat cheese is an option. English muffins with nut butters or organic jams are a great choice, or you can introduce mini pizzas in the morning by spreading pasta sauce on an English muffin, grating cheese on it, and popping it under the broiler or in the toaster oven.

Dairy

Ideally, you want to offer a half cup or its equivalent of dairy to toddlers and preschoolers in the morning, whether it's milk, yogurt or cheese. You can easily blend up a smoothie with a hand blender, standing blender or a food processor. Additions of fresh fruit, yogurts, and a splash of juice are exactly why most kids love the rich, creamy texture.

Protein

Nut butters like peanut, almond or cashew are a great choice for protein, as is cheese. You can offer animal proteins at breakfast in the form of meatballs, burgers, steak, sausages, and bacon, but, for busy families on the go, these are usually weekend breakfast foods. Toddlers can have cut up slices of ham or turkey cubes, or leftover chicken or drumsticks from the night before.

Eggs are a wholesome source of protein, and there are a million different things you can do with them. Try scrambling them and putting them in a warm tortilla with some grated cheese. This is a good option if you have a child on the run.

In the Know

According to a study published in the *Journal of Adolescent Health*, only one in five children consumes the recommended daily servings of fruit and vegetables, which are essential in delivering the necessary vitamins and nutrients for good health.[14] Most kids like fruit because it is sweet and tasty, and breakfast is a great time of day to offer these choices. In some European countries, cheese and vegetables are offered with whole grain breads for breakfast.

Spending a little time on the weekends to prepare a week or two of healthy food items you can store away in the freezer or fridge will help. Things like sheet pan meals are a great way to help you meal prep. Sheet pan meals make kitchen tasks much less complicated; all you need to do is toss all of your delicious healthy ingredients onto one sheet pan, bake them up, and then divide the portions among the family or pack them in snack bags. In less than thirty minutes, you can have a week's worth of meals prepared on one or two pans. Portion and seal airtight or freeze until needed.

Let's Review

As a parent, with or without a picky eater in your home, shopping, cooking and preparing meals can be somewhat challenging. I don't know many parents who have surplus hours to cook the picturesque, relaxing meals once enjoyed in our pre-parenting existence. Cooking methodically is a luxury more than a necessity these days, and could possibly be compared to enjoying a hobby. Your immediate family grows as children arrive and, before you realize, there seems to be an organic shift in lifestyle.

Clearly there are more responsibilities and many gears that need to be prioritized. If you or your partner works outside the home, you are a single parent, or you have multiple people to care for, including a picky or selective eater, chances are that

---

14   Tami M. Videon, Carolyn K. Manning, "Influences on adolescent eating patterns: the importance of family meals," *Journal of Adolescent Health* 32, no. 5 (May 2003): 365-373.

you are not busting out three-course, fancy meals like the good old days. Now, you undoubtedly don't have loads of time to grocery shop. Family meals certainly are not always easy, but they're always worth the effort and can help your picky eater. Many recipes in the chapters to come are designed with you in mind as well as your picky eater.

I certainly appreciate how hard it can seem to get a well-balanced meal on the table during busy nights juggling sports, dance class, homework, work and school events; I have been there. While zigzagging this path, as a professional chef I still struggled getting healthy, wholesome food on the table every day—especially three meals a day. Not to mention wading through the surplus of other duties such as homework and bath time.

Recognizing the level of responsibility you assume, I've selected recipes for this book that support your goal of getting good food on the table with a minimal number of steps. I want to support your already overextended roster rather than create additional effort for you. Eating as a family is truly soothing, for everyone—toddlers, teens and adults. Family meals can become a treasured ritual for everyone. If you don't make it happen every day, don't worry; lose the guilt. Make the most of your family meals when they occur.

Planning is essential; develop systems that make shopping, preparing, cooking and cleanup easier. Keep things simple. Family meals don't need to be elaborate to be healthy and effective.

Share the work. Enlist help from everyone in the family, from planning the shopping list to making lunches, bagging snacks, setting the table, pouring drinks, and cleaning up, removing the trash and sweeping the floor. This will make the load of having a picky eater easier too. Include your picky eater in all these responsibilities.

I cannot stress enough how preparing double batches when you're less rushed really helps cut down on time. Cook once; eat twice. This will ensure you can stay on track feeding your picky eater on your new regime instead of falling back into fast food or old habits just because they are convenient and you don't have anything on hand. Always stock healthy foods so you have them on hand. Stock your freezer or pantry and eat from here on busy weeknights.

Turn off technology, and tune into each other. Begin conversation during family meals, but keep it light. The dinner table is not the place for discipline. Balance family meals with simple vegetable side dishes, and fruit and yogurt for desserts.

The family meal does not have to be dinner; breakfast or lunch may work better in some households. Go with your family's flow, not societal norms. Offer your family one meal that includes all five food groups and everyone should be able to find something they'll want to eat.

Chapter Thirteen

BREAKFAST RECIPES

Green Eggs and Ham

This recipe is a natural, healthy way to color your eggs green. Pine nuts are traditional in a basil pesto but can be difficult to source, not to mention very expensive. Many people substitute with walnuts, which inherently have a bolder, somewhat bitter flavor iffy for picky eaters; instead, I use almonds due to the sweetness of the nut. This recipe was written for my children based off the book *Green Eggs and Ham* by the beloved Dr. Seuss. Share the book; make the dish.

You'll Need

8 eggs, cracked and lightly beaten

2–3 tablespoons prepared basil pesto

¾ cup pancetta or good quality ham, diced small

Freshly ground black pepper

1–2 tablespoons butter

Basil Pesto

4 cups fresh basil leaves, packed

1 cup fresh parsley, stems removed

2 cloves garlic, cleaned and coarsely chopped

1/2 cup pine nuts or almonds

1/2 cup Parmesan cheese, grated

1/2 teaspoon Himalayan or kosher salt

¼ teaspoon freshly ground black pepper

½ cup extra virgin olive oil

Juice of 1 lemon

Here's How

Basil Pesto

To the bowl of your food processor, add the garlic and pulse until minced. Add the nuts, Parmesan, salt and pepper. Process until the nuts are finely crushed, about 1 minute. Add the basil leaves, parsley, oil and lemon juice and pulse for an additional minute, until smooth.

Transfer the pesto to a sterilized jar with a tight-fitting lid. Pour a thin layer of olive oil on top of the pesto and seal tightly.

Makes approximately 2 cups

~Refrigerate up to 10 days or freeze up to 3 months.

~Time-Saving Tip: Many people also place the pesto into ice cube trays to freeze. Once frozen, remove individual cubes and place in an airtight container. Freezing individual portions saves time when cooking midweek. Use as needed.

Green Eggs and Ham

In a medium bowl, whisk the eggs. Add the ham, salt and pepper to taste. In a large nonstick skillet over medium heat, melt the butter and swirl to coat the bottom of the skillet. When the butter foams, add the egg mixture all at once. Let it set for about a minute. With a rubber spatula, stirring, begin moving the egg mixture around until light, fluffy and almost dry, about 3 to 5 minutes depending on your heat source. The last minute of cooking, while the eggs are still a little runny, add the basil pesto and work it into the eggs. Do not overcook.

Makes approximately 8 servings

~An umami recipe

~Omit nuts if you have an allergy or a picky texture eater

Sausage and Egg Muffins

These delicious umami sausage muffins are great for busy on-the-go families. You can use a 12-cup muffin tin and make enough for your freezer. You can also use a 6-cup muffin tin and trim the recipe in half.

You'll Need

6 slices whole wheat bread, for 12 rounds cut same size as the bottom of the muffin tin

1 cup Parmesan cheese, shredded

12 sausage links, cooked and crumbled

10 eggs, cracked and lightly beaten

1 bundle chives, finely chopped

¼ cup milk or milk substitute

2 tablespoons Worcestershire sauce

Kosher Salt and freshly ground black pepper

Healthy cooking spray

Here's How

Preheat your oven to 350 °F. Lightly spray muffin tins with nonstick cooking spray. I prefer to use a healthy cooking spray. Saves time on greasing the pan and makes cleanup easier too.

Using a cookie cutter or a child's plastic drinking cup, cut out two rounds per slice of bread, trying to cut them the same size as the bottom of the muffin pan. Place the bread rounds into the bottom of the prepared muffin pan. Set aside. Divide the cooked, crumbled sausage equally among the bread-lined muffin cups. Whisk the eggs, milk, onion powder, and garlic salt together. Add half the cheese to the egg mixture and mix again to combine. Add salt and fresh ground pepper.

Pour the egg mixture into the cups to cover fillings, about three-fourths full. Add scallions or chives and top with the remaining cheese. Bake for 15 minutes or until they are firm when poked with a fork, then cool completely. Store the muffins in the refrigerator in an airtight container until ready to use. Microwave or reheat in a toaster oven, and you're out the door! Delicious cold.

Makes 12 muffins

~An umami recipe

~Variation: For a lower carb meal you can completely omit the bread. Add your family's favorite vegetables, proteins, or anything you have left over.

~Freeze airtight safely up to 1 month.

Cloud Puffed Eggs

Cloud puffed eggs are a culinary staple in egg cookery. They are perfect for a surprise breakfast treat. Great for celebration breakfasts!

You'll Need

4 large eggs

Himalayan or kosher salt

Freshly ground black pepper

1/2 cup Parmesan cheese, finely grated

3 tablespoons chives, finely chopped, for garnish

Here's How

Preheat your oven to 400 °F. Line a baking sheet with parchment paper or a silicon baking mat. Set aside.

Separate the egg whites from the egg yolks by placing the whites in a large mixing bowl and the yolks in a small bowl, careful not to break them. Set yolks aside.

Using a whisk or a hand mixer, beat the egg whites until stiff peaks form. Gently fold in Parmesan cheese and season the egg whites with salt and pepper. Create four mounds of egg whites on a baking sheet lined with parchment paper. Indent the centers of each to look like nests.

Bake until slightly golden and the egg whites become sturdy, about 3 minutes. Carefully add each egg yolk to the center of each egg white "cloud." Season the yolk with salt and pepper. Bake until the yolks are just set, about 3 additional minutes.

Makes 4 servings

~Variations: Add chopped cooked pancetta, crumbled bacon, diced ham, small-chopped red bell peppers, scallions, or any of your favorite breakfast foods to the egg whites after they have stiff peaks to make this an umami recipe. Be extra careful not to deflate the whites when folding in.

Egg Treasure Muffins

These muffins are great for grab and go days. A little bit of work, but the outcome is worth it. When you bite into this delicious, savory muffin, a treasure is revealed. Kids love seeing a whole cooked egg inside. This recipe must be made with a jumbo-size muffin tin because the regular muffin tins are not large enough to hold the complete egg and the batter. You can find these larger muffin tins at any cookware supply store or order them online.

You'll Need

7 organic eggs

6 strips nitrate-free bacon, cut into ¼-inch strips

3/4 cup buttermilk

1/2 cup full fat plain Greek yogurt

2 tablespoons olive oil

1 cup cheddar cheese, grated

1/2 cup Parmesan cheese, finely grated

1 cup scallions, chopped

1/2 teaspoon kosher salt

1/4 teaspoon ground cayenne pepper

1/2 teaspoon freshly ground black pepper

1 1/2 cups all-purpose flour

1 teaspoon baking powder

1/4 teaspoon baking soda

Here's How

Preheat your oven to 350 °F. Spray a jumbo six-cup muffin pan with quality nonstick cooking spray. Set aside. Heat a 10-inch nonstick pan over medium heat. Add bacon pieces and cook until lightly browned but not cooked through. Remove onto a paper towel and set aside.

In a large mixing bowl, sift together the flour, baking soda, baking powder, salt, pepper and cayenne. Mix to combine. Set aside. In an additional bowl, combine 1 egg, buttermilk, olive oil, and yogurt, and whisk to combine. Slowly add the wet ingredients into the dry ingredients while whisking continuously to prevent lumps. Once combined, fold in the cheese, bacon and scallions.

Do not overmix. Inside the prepared muffin tin, place approximately 4 tablespoons of the muffin batter in the bottom of each cup. Bang the muffin tin on your work surface to level the batter. With the back of a wet spoon, make a round indentation in the batter deep enough to hold an egg.

Gently crack an egg into a small measuring cup or a gravy spoon, and then position the raw egg in the indentation in the muffin batter. If you are feeling brave, you can crack the egg right into the tin. Once you have placed all your raw eggs in the tins, divide the remaining batter on top of the eggs to cover. This little step will help keep the egg in place.

Bake your muffins on a sheet pan for 20–25 minutes until golden brown. Remove from oven and allow the muffins to rest for 5 minutes before turning out onto a cooling rack. Serve warm or cold.

Makes 6 large muffins

~ *An umami recipe*

~*Variation: Add your family's favorite vegetables, proteins or anything you have left over.*

~*Do not freeze. Refrigerate airtight safely up to 1 week.*

~*Time-Saving Tip: Using a wet spoon will keep the dough from sticking to the spoon. This technique will allow you to work quickly without creating a sticky mess*

Ham and Cheese Breakfast Pie

Breakfast is less complicated when you can toss all of your ingredients onto one sheet pan, bake it up, and then divide it among your family. This is an easy dish you can prepare the night before and pop in the oven first thing in the morning. Make it, bake it, and reheat it on your way out the door.

You'll Need

1 recipe homemade pizza dough or healthy premade dough from your grocer

3 tablespoons butter, divided

12 large eggs

1/4 cup half and half, cream, or whole milk

1/4 cup chives or scallions, finely chopped (optional)

1/2 pound nitrate-free ham, thinly sliced

12 slices real cheddar cheese

1 teaspoon kosher salt

1 teaspoon freshly ground pepper

1 teaspoon everything bagel seasoning (optional)

Your favorite cooking spray

Here's How

Preheat oven to 375 °F. Prepare a 9 x 13-inch sheet pan with cooking spray. Divide the pizza dough in half. Fit a portion of pizza dough into the prepared sheet pan. This takes some wrestling. Roll out the additional portion of dough to fit on top. Allow to rest if the dough is snapping back to its original shape, and begin again in a minute or two. Cover with a clean dishtowel and set aside.

In a large bowl, whisk together the eggs, cream, salt and pepper. In a large, nonstick pan over medium heat, melt half the butter. When the butter is foamy, reduce heat to low and add the egg mixture. Cook the egg mixture, stirring often with a rubber spatula, until the eggs are almost set but still moist. Taste. Adjust the seasoning with salt and pepper, and remove from the heat. Add a layer of ham to the pizza dough in the pan, and then top with the scrambled eggs, chives and grated cheese.

Top with the second portion of pizza dough, pinching the borders shut to seal. Melt remaining butter in microwave. Brush melted butter on top of dough, and then sprinkle with everything bagel seasoning. Make a few slits with a knife here and there to vent steam, and bake until golden brown, about 25 to 30 minutes.

If the dough is browning too quickly, cover with foil. Allow the pie to cool for at least 15 minutes before slicing into squares. Serve warm.

Makes approximately 6 servings

~*An umami recipe*

~*Variation: Add your family's favorite vegetables, proteins, or anything you have left over.*

~*Freeze airtight safely up to 1 month.*

~*Time-Saving Tip: If you are preparing this the night before, make sure you keep the complete sheet pan sealed airtight and in the refrigerator overnight to prevent the dough from doubling.*

Breakfast Frittata

I know how busy mornings can be as a parent. You undoubtedly have no extra time on your hands. Making a frittata the night before makes life in the morning less frantic—if that's at all possible. With a precooked frittata, you can grab a slice and heat it in the microwave or serve it cold in less than five minutes. The best part is that you don't really need a recipe, and you can also eat these for lunch or dinner.

Start by cooking your proteins, like bacon, ham cubes or sausages. You can use any ingredients you want—you can also completely skip animal proteins. Add the vegetables and cook over medium heat in a little oil, or the fat from the meat if you included it.

After a minute or so of sautéing your veggies, add chopped garlic and shallots. Add 8 eggs that have been slightly whipped with cream and seasoned with salt and pepper. At this point, you can toss in delicate baby spinach leaves and add some fine-grated cheese and chopped herbs. Continue to cook in the pan for an additional 5 minutes until the eggs pull away from the sides of the pan. Place the whole oven-safe skillet into a 350 °F oven for about 15 to 20 minutes, or until the eggs are cooked through. The frittata will be firm to the touch and a light, toasty brown when it's ready.

Frittata can be served immediately warm or cooled and then chilled. Top with sour cream, salsa, or guacamole, or serve plain. Any 10-inch oven-safe skillet is a perfect size for an 8-egg frittata. For a classic look, bake your masterpiece in a cast-iron skillet. Larger dimensions will work but will yield thinner frittatas and require less cooking time.

~Refrigerate airtight safely up to 1 week.

The Picky Eater's Pizza Frittata

You'll Need

3 tablespoons olive oil

1 tablespoon butter

1/2 onion, very finely chopped

1 clove garlic, finely minced

1 cup nitrate-free Italian sausage or pepperoni, diced small

8 eggs, cracked and lightly whipped

2 tablespoons homemade pasta sauce

1 tablespoon Worcestershire or Asian fish sauce

1/2 cup milk

1/2 cup Parmesan cheese, grated, and additional cheese for topping

1/4 cup black olives, sliced

1/2 teaspoon kosher salt

1/2 teaspoon freshly ground pepper

Here's How

Preheat the oven to 350 °F. In a 10-inch oven-safe skillet, heat the oil and the butter. Add the diced onions and sauté until translucent, about 3 minutes. Add the diced sausage and sauté until browned, about 3 to 5 minutes. Add the garlic and toss to cook an additional minute. While the sausage is browning, whisk the milk, pasta sauce and Parmesan cheese together with the eggs. Season with salt, pepper, Worcestershire or fish sauce to create an umami experience.

Add egg mixture to the preheated skillet and cook on low heat until the eggs begin to pull away from the pan, about 5 to 8 minutes. Top with black olives and additional cheese. Place the entire oven-safe skillet into the preheated oven for about 15 to 18 minutes. Serve warm or cold with homemade ketchup.

Makes approximately 10–12 servings

~ *An umami recipe*

~*Variation: Add your family's favorite vegetables, proteins or anything you have left over.*

~*Freeze airtight safely up to 1 month. Refrigerate airtight safely up to 1 week.*

Homemade Ketchup

This recipe is in the breakfast section because my children put ketchup on their breakfast scrambles in the morning. Maybe yours will too. Making homemade ketchup will yield a delicious thick tomato condiment that is richer and more rustic in flavor than commercial brands and without artificial ingredients and shelf stabilizers. Be sure to make this with your child; he will be amazed—not to mention this recipe is high in umami.

You'll Need

2 tablespoons good quality olive oil

1 medium onion, diced large

1 clove garlic, chopped

1 (28-ounce) can tomato puree

1/2 cup brown sugar

1/4 cup apple cider vinegar

1 tablespoon tomato paste

1 teaspoon kosher salt

1/2 teaspoon ground mustard

1/8 teaspoon ground cloves

1/4 teaspoon ground allspice

1 tablespoon crushed red pepper

1/2 teaspoon ground cayenne pepper

Here's How

Heat oil in a pot over medium heat. Sauté the onion for 5 to 8 minutes until translucent. Add the garlic and stir together. Add the tomato puree, brown sugar, vinegar, tomato paste, salt, mustard, cloves, allspice, red pepper flakes and cayenne pepper, and stir to combine. Increase heat to high and bring to a boil, then reduce heat to low and simmer, stirring occasionally, for 45 to 60 minutes until it is thick like ketchup. With an immersion blender, food processor or standing blender, puree the mixture until smooth. Adjust seasonings if needed, and pour ketchup into an airtight container and seal.

Makes approximately 4 cups

~An umami recipe

~Refrigerate for up to 1 month.

Maddox Go-Go Cones

My kids couldn't wait for breakfast when we had Go-Go Cones. I prefer to use regular organic, non-sugar cones. This is a great way to take breakfast on the go. Fill the cones with anything the kids will eat. I usually filled ours with scrambled eggs, sausage and breakfast potatoes topped with cheese, but the kids loved when I filled them with frozen yogurts and let them pick their own toppings.

You'll Need

Store-bought organic ice cream cones

Yogurt that has been frozen a minimum of an hour

Fresh fruit

Fresh fruit smoothie

Granola, seeds, or nuts

Honey or lite maple syrup

Cinnamon

Here's How

Place slightly frozen yogurt in the bottom of the cone, top with fresh fruit, additional yogurt and top with healthy cereals, granolas, nuts or seeds of your child's choice.

~Variations: Top with scrambled eggs and bacon and cheese or oatmeal with granola and sliced banana toppings. Use cottage cheese instead of yogurt, or add last night's leftovers.

Traditional Breakfast Fillings

Egg-whites scramble

Scrambled eggs and bacon with cheese

Scrambled eggs and diced ham with cheese

Egg, sausage, and cheese scramble

Cooked oatmeal, honey, peanut butter, and bananas

Cooked oatmeal, almond butter, maple syrup, and sliced apples

Tossed Cobb salad

Mozzarella, basil, and tomatoes, tossed in lite vinaigrette

Lettuce, small cubed cheese, sliced black olives

Egg salad

Tuna salad

Hummus and shredded carrots

Turkey, cheese, mustard, and lettuce

Any prepared meals your family enjoys can be filled and served in a Go-Go Cone. Make a pizza cone by layering fresh grated cheese and healthy tomato sauce, combined with any of your child's favorite pizza toppings. Layer throughout the cone and add extra cheese to the top off the cone. Place your filled pizza go-cones in an oven-safe coffee mug, bakeware, or a specialized rack that can hold them upright. Warm the cones for a minute or two until the cheese is melted and cones are warmed through. Fillings are limitless.

Dinner for Breakfast Go-Go Cones

Go-go taco cones

Go-go mashed potato and meatloaf cones

Mac and cheese cones

Philly cheesesteak cones

Chicken pot pie cones

Caesar salad cones

Dutch Baby Pancake

A Dutch baby is a popover-like pancake that kids love for its taste but also for the way it looks. A Dutch baby is a wacky, puffed-up, giant balloon that collapses straight from the oven. It's also called a German pancake or a Bismarck. Although it's traditionally made with sautéed apples, it is most commonly made without fruit. I love to make ours with blueberries, which are a great antioxidant, but I notice that picky eaters love this with bananas.

You'll Need

3 large eggs, room temperature

½ cup whole milk or substitute

½ cup all-purpose flour or whole wheat

¼ teaspoon kosher salt

2 tablespoons unsalted butter

2 ripe bananas, sliced

1 tablespoon organic all-natural maple syrup or honey

½ teaspoon ground cinnamon

Here's How

Preheat the oven to 425 °F. In a small mixing bowl, combine the eggs and milk. Whisk without overbeating, or the eggs will deflate in the oven. Add the flour, salt, and cinnamon, and whisk out any lumps. Set aside.

Place an oven-safe, 10-inch skillet on the stove, and turn the heat to medium. Add the butter and, when it is hot, add the bananas, making sure the slices are in a single layer and not crowded on top of one another, and do not overcook.

Add maple syrup and cook until brown and sticky, about 3 minutes. Add the egg mixture and cook on high for an additional 1 minute. Carefully move the hot skillet to the oven and complete the cooking process. Bake for about 20 minutes until puffy and almost dry. Turn off the oven and allow the Dutch baby to sit undisturbed in the oven for an additional 5 minutes.

Remove from the oven and serve immediately with warmed maple syrup or honey. You can also dust with a slight amount of powdered sugar if your picky eater is not living sugar free.

Makes approximately 2 to 4 servings

~Variations: Use any fruit your child desires, or prepare plain

Nut Milk Pancakes

You'll go nuts over these cashew milk pancakes. For cake-like pancakes, reduce the amount of cashew milk; for thinner pancakes, add additional milk. These are great for kids that need an animal milk alternative. Works with rice and soy milk also. Use your child's favorite compound butters for topping these delicious pancakes.

You'll Need

2 cups whole wheat or all-purpose flour

2 tablespoons monk fruit sugar granules or organic cane sugar

1/2 teaspoon Himalayan or kosher salt

1½ tablespoons baking powder

2 large eggs, well beaten

1/4 cup extra virgin non-flavored coconut oil or butter, melted

2 cups favorite nut or cow's milk, room temperature

1 teaspoon flavored essential oil or extract of your choice (I use hazelnut or vanilla)

Your favorite cooking spray

Here's How

Sift together the flour, sugar, salt and baking powder. Make a well in the center of the flour. Add the beaten eggs, cashew milk and melted butter. Whisk to combine until smooth and lump free. Heat a pan over medium-low. Use your favorite healthy cooking spray to continuously maintain a nonstick surface. If your pan begins to smoke, turn the heat down.

Ladle 2 to 3 ounces of the batter in the pan with a ladle. Using the back of the ladle, create circular motions from the center out. This will help you maintain a good round pancake shape. Cook about 2 minutes until bubbles form and the edges turn brown. Flip and continue to cook another 1 to 2 minutes, or until golden.

Makes approximately 8 to 10 pancakes

~Time-Saving Tip: Make a double batch for midweek grab-and-go meals. Individually frozen pancakes can be reheated in the toaster.

Hula Hoop Waffles with Tropical Salsa

You'll Need

2 eggs

1/3 cup butter or coconut oil, melted

1¾ cups milk or favorite substitute

2 cups flour

2 tablespoons sugar or healthy sugar substitute

4 teaspoons baking powder

1/2 teaspoon salt

1 teaspoon vanilla extract

1/2 cup flaked coconut (optional)

Tropical Fruit Salsa (see recipe on the right)

Warm maple syrup or honey, for topping

Here's How

Preheat a waffle iron and spray it lightly with nonstick cooking spray. In a medium bowl, whisk together the flour, sugar, baking powder and salt. Set aside. In an additional bowl, whisk the eggs until foamy; add the melted butter and milk to the egg mixture. Combine the wet ingredients to the dry ingredients while smoothing out any lumps. Fold in the flaked coconut if you are using it.

Pour just enough batter to fill the well of the waffle iron, close the lid, and bake until the steam ends and the waffle is lightly browned and crisp, about 3 to 4 minutes. Remove the waffle and repeat with the remaining batter. Serve with warm maple syrup on the side and tropical fruit salsa.

Makes approximately 8 to 10 waffles

~Time-Saving Tip: Individual frozen waffles can be frozen up to 1 month and reheated in the toaster on busy mornings

Tropical Fruit Salsa

My whole family loves tropical salsas on waffles. Even though I do have a picky eater, I have additional family members that love this recipe. My picky eater ironically loved anything with a serrano chili. If your child prefers foods without heat, remove the chili and the onion until her palate develops a little more as she matures. This is a fun fruit salsa the family will enjoy.

You'll Need

1 large ripe mango, diced small

1 cup pineapple, diced small

1 kiwi, peeled, diced small

1/4 cup chives, finely chopped

1/2 purple onion, diced very small

1/2 cup sweet red bell pepper, diced very small

1/4 cup parsley, finely minced

1/4 cup cilantro, minced

2–3 teaspoons rice or apple cider vinegar

1/4 teaspoon Kosher salt

Juice and zest of 1 lime

1–2 tablespoons warm honey to taste

1/2 serrano chili, minced (optional)

Here's How

Combine all ingredients in a bowl, toss, and chill. Serve close to room temperature. Try this salsa with your favorite tortilla chips, too!

Makes approximately 2 cups

~Time-Saving Tip: Make up to 1 day in advance

Vegan Pumpkin Donuts

Topped with cinnamon sugar, these vegan pumpkin donuts are delicious, won't stick around long, and are easy to make. I usually don't like to serve sugar-leading foods to the kids, but as a once-in-a-while treat, this recipe is about as healthy as we're going to get with a donut. You can also use organic, naturally occurring sugar substitutes like stevia. One thing you can count on with this recipe is there are no additional artificial ingredients like you might find in a packaged, store-bought breakfast treat.

You'll Need

2½ cups cake flour, sifted

3/4 cup light brown sugar, packed

1 teaspoon salt

2 teaspoon baking powder

1/2 cup canned or fresh pumpkin puree

1/4 teaspoon ground allspice

4 heaping tablespoons coconut oil or vegan butter, melted

1 cup almond milk

Cinnamon sugar coating

Cinnamon Sugar Coating

6 teaspoons extra virgin coconut oil or vegan butter, melted

1 1/2 cup organic sugar, for dusting

1/4 cup ground cinnamon

Here's How

Generously grease a donut pan. Set aside on top of a foil-lined cookie sheet. Preheat the oven to 350 °F. In a large bowl, sift the dry ingredients together, or whisk to remove any lumps. In a separate bowl, whisk together the pumpkin puree, coconut oil, and almond milk.

Gently fold the wet mixture into the dry mixture. Stir to combine. Do not overmix. Spoon mixture into the prepared donut pan and bake for about 10 to 12 minutes, or until the donuts spring back when lightly pressed. While cooling the donuts, prepare the toppings.

In a medium saucepan, melt the coconut oil. Set aside. In a bowl or casserole baking dish, combine the sugar and cinnamon. Set aside. Once the donuts are cool enough to handle, quickly dip them in the melted coconut oil, and then roll them in the cinnamon sugar mixture. Shake off any excess cinnamon sugar.

Makes approximately 1 dozen donuts

~*Variation: You can also use pumpkin pie spice in place of cinnamon.*

Billy Goat Breakfast Biscuits

A high-carb meal for those little ones that are burning lots of energy first thing in the morning!

You'll Need

8–10 turkey sausages or favorite links

1½ tablespoons olive oil

1 cup yellow potatoes, diced small

1/2 cup green onions, thinly sliced

1 teaspoon garlic, minced

8 eggs, beaten

1/2 cup cheddar cheese, grated

1/4 teaspoon salt

Freshly ground black pepper

8–10 **Billy Goat Biscuits** (see recipe below)

Here's How

Preheat the oven to 350 °F. Place a 10-inch ovenproof skillet over medium heat and cook sausages. Remove the sausages to a plate and cut into bite-size pieces. Set aside. In the same skillet, over medium heat, warm the oil and add the potatoes. Sauté the potatoes until tender, about 5 to 8 minutes, add onions, and cook until translucent. Return the sausage back to the pan and continue to brown all the ingredients for an additional 3 to 5 minutes.

In a medium bowl, whisk together the eggs, garlic, cheese, salt and pepper to taste. Pour the egg mixture over the sausage and potato mixture in the skillet. Stir to combine until the eggs are set, about 5 minutes.

Split warm biscuits, fill with the egg scramble, and wrap in parchment paper or foil for a grab-and-go meal. You can also enjoy this biscuit recipe on its own with delicious compound butter or flavored cream cheese.

Makes approximately 8 to 10 servings.

~Time-Saving Tip: Fill biscuits, wrap individually and freeze. Thaw and reheat on the go. Individually-made biscuits filled with scrambled egg mixtures can be reheated in the toaster oven or microwave.
~Freeze up to 2 weeks airtight.

Billy Goat Biscuits

You'll Need

3 cups all-purpose flour

1 tablespoon salt

1½ teaspoons baking powder

1 teaspoon sugar

1/2 teaspoon salt

6 tablespoons unsalted butter, cold

1 cup buttermilk

Here's How

Preheat the oven to 425 °F. In a large bowl, or a plastic food storage bag for easy cleanup, combine the flour, baking powder, baking soda, sugar and salt. Using your fingers, cut the butter into the flour mixture until it resembles coarse crumbs. Work quickly so you don't warm the butter with your body temperature. The secret to flaky dough is to use cold ingredients and not to overwork the dough.

Once your mixture resembles the size of small peas, add the buttermilk all at once and stir with your hand until the mixture holds together. Do not overmix. Gather the dough into a ball, turn it onto a lightly-floured surface, and knead for about 30 seconds. Pat the dough into a rectangle about ¾ of an inch thick. Fold it into thirds like a letter and roll gently with a floured rolling pin until the dough is 3/4 of an inch thick again. Cut into circles with a biscuit cutter for traditional round biscuits.

Place the biscuits on a prepared baking sheet, one inch apart. Brush the tops of the biscuits with milk to assist with browning. Place in the preheated oven and bake until puffed up and slightly browned. About 18 to 20 minutes.

Makes approximately 1 dozen mini biscuits

~Variations: Serve with honey butter, your favorite compound butter, or flavored cream cheeses. These biscuits make a

great base for breakfast sandwiches or accompanying a great breakfast.

~Time-Saving Tip: Roll the dough into a rectangle and then cut into squares. Store airtight; biscuits will keep up to 1 week on your counter. Gently reheat before serving.

Cinnamon Honey Compound Butter

If you've been looking for a way to renovate a few of your recipes but don't want to put a lot of time and effort into it, look no further than compound butter. Compound butters are essentially butter with the addition of fresh herbs, aromatics, or other flavors. Compound butters prove there is a way to make foods taste amazing with less effort. You can combine fresh fruit, honey, and ground spices, too. Delicious on sandwiches, toasted bagels, baked potatoes, warm biscuits, or grilled foods. Try any combinations your family will love. You can also make the same additions to cream cheese.

You'll Need

1 stick unsalted butter, room temperature

1–2 tablespoons honey

1/2 teaspoon ground cinnamon

Here's How

Combine butter and honey in a small bowl or food processor. blend until well combined. Add cinnamon; blend throughout the butter. Place the butter on a sheet of parchment paper or plastic wrap, and roll it into a log, sealing the wrap tightly around the butter. Chill the log until firm and then slice into coins to use, or place in a wide-mouth glass jar and seal airtight.

Makes approximately 4 ounces of flavored butter

A Note on Flavored Butters and Cream Cheese Spreads

Once you understand the method for making compound butters, you can also make cream cheese spreads, an easy process that will supply you with an endless variety of flavors you and your family will love. Begin with plain, softened cream cheese or butter at room temperature. Add your favorite ingredients and mix well. Place the flavored cream cheeses and butters in airtight containers such as wide-mouth glass Mason jars. Always keep refrigerated and serve chilled.

I'm sharing fun, sweet, and savory recipes throughout to get you started. These are interchangeable between butter and cream cheese. Remember to keep sugary foods to a minimum. Have fun and use your imagination. You might want to gather a few flavor suggestions from your child and allow her to help you prepare them.

Savory compound butter combinations are also perfect for accompanying grilled foods, steamed vegetables, or warm breakfast egg scrambles. And if your child requests dinner for breakfast, compound butters can enhance flavor. Start out using 8 ounces of butter or cream cheese.

Savory Garlic and Olive Oil Butter

Keep in mind that the garlic in this recipe is raw, so, to use this recipe effectively, you should cook with it. This recipe is the perfect compound butter for tossing with fresh steamed vegetables, scrambled eggs or cooked pasta.

You'll Need

8 ounces unsalted organic butter, room temperature

1 teaspoon good quality extra virgin olive oil

1 tablespoon fresh shallot, finely minced

1 small clove garlic, finely minced or pressed

1 tablespoon fresh herbs of your choice, chopped

1/4 teaspoon kosher salt

Here's How

Combine garlic, shallots, and herbs in a food processor and pulse until chopped fine. Add olive oil and salt. Blend throughout the butter. Place the butter on a sheet of parchment paper or plastic wrap, roll it into a log, sealing the wrap tightly around the butter, and chill the log until firm, or place in a glass jar with a tight lid.

Makes approximately 1 cup

Cinnamon-Date Cream Cheese

This is a great sweet recipe made with the impressive benefits of medjool dates, which help with normal growth and development. They will be great for everyone in the family, and a natural way to sweeten.

You'll Need

8 ounces cream cheese, softened

1/2 cup medjool dates, packed

1/2 teaspoon ground cinnamon

Here's How

In the bowl of your food processor, add the dates and pulse until a sticky paste appears. Add the cinnamon and cream cheese. Pulse until the dates and cinnamon are swirled throughout. Spoon mixture into a glass jar with a tight lid, keep refrigerated, and serve chilled. This is tasty on morning bagels.

Makes approximately 1 cup

Warm Waffle Sammies with Bananas and Almond and Strawberry Butters

This is a hearty breakfast sandwich full of flavor! If you have a picky eater opposing textured foods and he complains about textures, substitute pancakes for waffles.

You'll Need

4 homemade waffles

4 tablespoons almond butter

4 tablespoons fresh strawberry compound butter (see **Strawberry and Vanilla Cream Cheese** recipe below)

Fresh banana slices

1/4 cup dried banana chip dust

Ground cinnamon to taste

Here's How

In the bowl of your food processor, blitz the dried banana chips into dust. Place in an airtight jar and set aside. Toast the waffles in a toaster or oven. Layer the waffle with almond butter, strawberry butter, and sliced bananas. Season with banana chip dust and a sprinkle of cinnamon, top with the other waffle, and press to sandwich together. Serve toasty warm.

Makes 2 servings

~Variations: Alternative fillings are okay to use. This is another great grab-and-go meal.

Strawberry and Vanilla Cream Cheese

You'll Need

16 ounces cream cheese, softened

10 fresh sweet strawberries, cleaned and hulled

1 tablespoon honey

1/2 teaspoon vanilla essential oil or natural extract, or the seeds scraped from one vanilla bean pod, vanilla bean pod reserved

Here's How

Slice your vanilla bean pod lengthwise without slicing in half. With a paring knife, scrape seeds out of the pod. Set the pod aside. Combine all your ingredients into the bowl of your food processor (except for vanilla bean pod). Blend until well combined. Place the cream cheese mixture into an airtight glass jar; place vanilla bean pod inside the butter in the container to continue flavoring. Refrigerate and serve cold.

Makes approximately 2 cups

Stone Fruit Oatmeal with Coconut Milk

You'll Need

    1½ cups water

    1 large fresh ripe but firm nectarine or peach, skin removed and diced medium, or substitute with tropical fruit if your child prefers

    1 cup rolled oats

    Pinch of salt

    Sprinkle of cinnamon

    1/4 cup warm coconut, rice, or almond milk

    1 tablespoon butter

    Toasted coconut, for garnish (optional)

Here's How

If you are toasting coconut, preheat the oven to 350 °F. Lay coconut flakes on nonstick baking tray, and place in the oven until brown. Bake for about 5 minutes depending on your oven. Shredded coconut will toast fast, so be careful not to burn it. Set aside to cool.

In a small saucepan, heat the water with salt. Bring to a boil. Add oatmeal and stir to combine. Cook over medium heat about 1 minute. Add the diced peaches, butter and cinnamon; stir to combine. Return to the stove, reduce heat and simmer until peaches are warmed through and desired consistency is reached, about 1 to 2 additional minutes.

Warm coconut milk in a separate saucepan while oats are cooking. When ready to serve, place oatmeal into bowls and top with warm coconut milk. Serve garnishes on the side and allow your child to top off her own breakfast bowls, or skip the coconut milk and load up a **Maddox Go-Go Cone** (see page 105).

Makes approximately 2 to 4 servings

Sliced Apple Donut Rings

You'll Need

12 ounces cream cheese, softened, cut into thirds

2 teaspoons organic honey, divided

1/2 cup warmed nut butter

1/4–1/2 teaspoon beetroot powder

3 apples

Assorted healthy toppings for decorating

Here's How

Divide cream cheese among three small bowls. In one bowl, add 1 teaspoon of the honey. In an additional bowl, add melted nut butter, and, in the last bowl, add remaining teaspoon of honey and the beetroot. Stir ingredients together in each bowl until combined. Core the apples and slice into ¼-inch to ½-inch discs. If you don't have an apple core tool, slice the apples in discs. Lay flat and remove the core with a 1-inch round cookie cutter to hollow out centers.

Spread mixtures on apple slices and sprinkle with assorted healthy toppings. Serve immediately.

Makes 4 to 6 servings

~Time-Saving Tip: Organic, dried beetroot powder can be purchased online and is a good natural food coloring.

French Toast Muffins

You'll Need

1 large brioche loaf, cut into 1-inch cubes (about 12 cups)

6 whole eggs

2 cups almond, coconut, soy, or cow's milk

1/2 cup extra virgin coconut oil, or vegan or regular organic butter, melted

1 cup stevia or organic sugar of your choice

1/2 cup organic brown sugar, packed

1 tablespoon vanilla extract

1/4 teaspoon ground nutmeg

1/2 teaspoon ground cinnamon

1/2 teaspoon kosher salt

1 apple, diced small

1 cup raisins, currants, or dried cherries (optional)

1 cup banana granola or your favorite organic granola

3 tablespoons stevia crystals or organic sugar for dusting

1 tablespoon ground cinnamon

Here's How

Preheat the oven to 350 °F. Spray a 12-cup muffin pan with nonstick spray, or use a nonstick silicon muffin pan. Place on a sheet pan and set aside.

In a large mixing bowl, combine all wet ingredients and seasonings; whisk well. Add cubed bread and toss to soak in the wet egg mixture for about 30 minutes. Toss again midway, ensuring all cubes become saturated. Gently fold in banana granola.

Without squeezing the cubed bread, gradually ladle or pour into each prepared muffin tin, and bake for approximately 45 minutes. After the first 25 minutes, combine 3 tablespoons of sugar with 1 tablespoon of cinnamon and sprinkle over the muffins. Return to oven. Bake 15 to 20 additional minutes.

Makes approximately 6 servings.

~Time-Saving Tip: Stevia is a sweetener and FDA-approved sugar substitute extracted from the leaves of the plant species Stevia Rebaudiana. *Found in most markets, or can be purchased online.*

Pumpkin Pie Pancakes with Bacon Maple Butter

This recipe is easy to make and best when made with fresh pumpkin or butternut squash puree. Pancakes won't be so orange with homemade puree, and the batter will result in a lighter, fluffier pancake. If pumpkins are not in season or you are short on time, use canned pumpkin.

You'll Need

1/2 cup pumpkin puree, canned or **Fresh Pumpkin Puree** (see recipe below)

1/4 cup low-fat vanilla yogurt

2 cups whole wheat or gluten-free flour

2 teaspoons baking powder

1 teaspoon baking soda

2 large eggs

4 tablespoons dark brown or coconut sugar

1/4 teaspoon Kosher salt

1 tablespoon ground cinnamon

1/4 teaspoon ground cloves

1/2 teaspoon ground ginger

1/2 teaspoon ground nutmeg

1 teaspoon vanilla extract

Healthy cooking spray

Maple syrup or honey, warmed

Bacon Maple Butter (see recipe below)

Here's How

In a large mixing bowl, combine the dry ingredients and set aside. In a medium mixing bowl, whisk together pumpkin, yogurt, eggs, sugar, and vanilla extract. Add the wet ingredients to the dry ingredients, and mix to combine. The batter will be inherently lumpy; do not overmix.

Heat a large nonstick skillet coated with healthy cooking spray over medium heat. With a ladle, portion 2 to 3 ounces of batter for each pancake into the warmed, prepared pan. With the back of the ladle, make a circular motion from the center out to make 4-to-5-inch pancakes.

Cook until bubbles emerge from the center of the pancake and the sides change from shiny to dull, approximately 3 to 5 minutes.

Quickly slide a spatula under the pancake and flip over. Continue to cook for an additional 2 to 3 minutes, or until golden brown. Top with bacon maple butter, warm syrup or warm honey.

Makes approximately 4 to 5 servings

~Time-Saving Tip: Make an additional recipe and freeze individual pancakes on a sheet tray. Once frozen, you can repack in an airtight container. Use the toaster to reheat during a midweek morning dash out the door.

Fresh Pumpkin or Squash Puree

Pumpkin or squash puree is very simple to make and is delicious in many recipes. It also freezes well. Ask your grocery expert for "pie pumpkins"—they are a sweeter variety of pumpkin, with great flavor. Some are seasonal. Many can be found year-round.

You'll Need

1 large pumpkin or squash (5–6 pounds)

2 tablespoons butter, softened

Here's How

Preheat oven to 375 °F. Place pumpkin on a damp dishtowel on a flat work surface. With a long, sharp, serrated knife, carefully saw the pumpkin in half, crosswise through the stem, and scoop out the seeds and strings. Keep the seeds to roast.

Butter the flesh and place pumpkin halves, cut-side down, onto an unlined baking sheet. Roast, uncovered, for 40 to 60 minutes, or until tender. Remove from the oven and allow the flesh to cool enough to handle.

When cool, carefully scrape the flesh from skin. Discard the skin. Using a food processor or blender, puree until velvety smooth. Store airtight until ready to use or freeze.

Makes approximately 3 to 4 cups puree

Bacon Maple Butter

This compound butter is a delicious pairing for my **Pumpkin Pie Pancakes** (see page 130).

You'll Need

4 ounces unsalted butter, room temperature

2 pieces thick-sliced bacon, cooked crisp and crumbled

1 tablespoon maple syrup

Here's How

Combine all ingredients in a small food processor and whip until combined. Or smash together with a fork until all ingredients are combined. Shape into a log on a piece of plastic wrap, roll up, and twist ends tight to form a firm log. Chill. You can also place this delicious compound butter in a wide-mouth glass jar and refrigerate.

Makes approximately 1/2 cup

~Time-Saving Tip: Bring compound butter to room temperature before using.

Bananarama Munkie Bread

You'll Need

2½ cups flour

1 teaspoon salt

2 teaspoons baking soda

1 cup cold butter, cut into chunks

2 cups sugar

2 cups ripe bananas, mashed (about 6 bananas)

3 eggs, slightly beaten

2 teaspoons vanilla

1 cup walnuts, coarsely chopped (optional)

Here's How

Preheat the oven to 350 °F. Grease and flour two 8 x 4 x 3-inch loaf pans. Sift together the flour, salt and baking soda in a bowl. Set aside. In the bowl of your standing mixer, cream together the butter and sugar until pale. Add the mashed bananas, eggs, vanilla and walnuts until just combined.

In increments, add the dry ingredients to the butter mixture; stir until the batter is just blended. Do not overmix. Gently fold in the nuts. Pour the batter into the prepared pans and bake on sheet pans for 50 to 60 minutes, or until a toothpick inserted in the center of a loaf comes out clean. Gently top with foil for the last 15 minutes of baking if the loaves begin to get to brown.

Remove the loaves from the oven and allow them to cool in the pans for about 5 minutes, and then turn them out on a cooling rack and let them cool completely. Chill before cutting and use a serrated knife for the cleanest cuts.

Makes 2 loaves

*~Variation: Dust the top with powdered sugar
  before slicing.*

Bananarama Munkie Breakfast Sammie

This breakfast sandwich is a favorite in my family. The kids love making the flavored cream cheeses while waiting for the toaster to caramelize the sliced bread.

You'll Need

2 (½-inch-thin) slices of **Bananarama Munkie Bread** (see recipe on the left)

2 tablespoons whipped or flavored cream cheese

1/4 fresh banana, sliced lengthwise

1/2 teaspoon honey or organic maple syrup

Here's How

Toast the slices of bananarama bread to your desired darkness and remove from the toaster. Cool slightly so that you can handle them. Spread whipped cream cheese on both slices, top the cream cheese with banana slices, and drizzle the banana slices with honey. Top with the remaining slice of bananarama munkie bread. Slice diagonally and serve.

~Variation: In summertime, I toast the bread on the outdoor grill if serving for lunch or dinner. And yes, the grill does fire up in the morning a few days per week.

Cinnamon Apple Muffins

You'll Need

1¾ cups white or regular whole wheat flour

1½ teaspoons baking powder

1 teaspoon ground cinnamon

½ teaspoon baking soda

½ teaspoon salt

1 Granny Smith apple, grated

1 Granny Smith apple, peeled, seeded, and diced into ¼-inch dice

⅓ cup coconut oil, melted

½ cup maple syrup or honey

2 eggs, room temperature

½ cup plain Greek yogurt

½ cup applesauce

1 teaspoon vanilla extract

Turbinado sugar to top muffins (optional)

Here's How

Preheat oven to 325 °F. Spray your 12-cup muffin tin with nonstick cooking spray. In a large mixing bowl, combine the flour, baking powder, cinnamon, baking soda and salt. Blend well with a whisk. Set aside.

In a medium mixing bowl, combine the coconut oil and warm maple syrup or honey. Beat on low speed. Add the eggs and continue to beat for 1 minute until eggs and oil combine.

Add yogurt, applesauce, diced and grated apples and vanilla. Mix well. Add the dry ingredients in a few additions and mix just until combined. Work quickly so the coconut oil does not begin to solidify. The batter will be very thick.

Divide the batter evenly between the muffin cups. Sprinkle the tops of the muffins with optional turbinado sugar. Bake muffins for 20 to 30 minutes, or until the muffins are golden on top and a toothpick inserted into a muffin comes out clean. Place the muffin tin on a cooling rack to cool. Store muffins in an airtight container.

Makes approximately 1 dozen

~Variations: Use any diced dry fruit your child will love. Make sure to reconstitute it by soaking in warm water for about 15 minutes.

Frozen Yogurt Bark

My children loved those frozen yogurt shops where you independently choose and dispense your chosen flavors into a serving container and add your own toppings, weigh it, and then pay for it. Making yogurt bark at home is similar but healthier and much more cost effective. This is great to serve for an occasional breakfast accompaniment or standing on its own. I also like to serve frozen yogurt bark for dessert.

You'll Need

2 cups whole milk plain Greek yogurt

3 tablespoons honey

1 teaspoon vanilla extract

A variety of toppings, from fruits to nuts

Here's How

Line a sheet pan with parchment or a silicon baking mat. Make sure the sheet pan can fit into your freezer lying flat. Set aside. In a small bowl, combine the yogurt, honey and vanilla. Spread onto the parchment-lined baking sheet in an even layer. Sprinkle with desired toppings and place in the freezer overnight. Simply break into pieces and serve.

~*Variations: Chocolate chips and raspberries, pistachios and pomegranate seeds, blueberries and slivered almonds, blackberries and granola, trail mix, diced mangos, kiwis and toasted coconut—the options are endless.*

Frozen Yogurt Bananas

Bananas and yogurt are a great pairing, and, if you need a new novelty for breakfast, serve a yogurt-dipped banana. What kid wouldn't eat this delicious treat for breakfast?

You'll Need

2 ripe bananas, halved

2 cups plain Greek yogurt

2 tablespoons fresh honey

4 popsicle sticks

Choice of toppings: dried fruit bits, mini chocolate chips, crushed banana chips, carob, cocoa, crumbled graham crackers, or nuts if your kids can have them

Here's How

Line a cookie sheet with parchment paper (again, one that can fit in your freezer—go make room now; you will thank me later).

Mix the yogurt with the honey in a gallon food-storage bag with the sides rolled back so you can get in and out of the bag— you know how I love no additional cleanup. Line an additional sheet pan with parchment and toppings of your choice. Set the topping tray to the right of the yogurt-filled bag and, next to the toppings, place the sheet pan ready for the freezer. Working from left to right, dunk the bananas in the honey yogurt, covering the entire banana by rolling it in the yogurt.

Remove, and gently shake excess yogurt off. Next, roll the bananas in the toppings and place on the freezer tray. Carefully insert the popsicle sticks, and place them all in the freezer for a minimum of 1 hour. Once frozen, wrap and seal individually, airtight. This treat is best consumed at the family table. The yogurt melts quickly without stabilizers and can become messy— not great for the car.

Makes approximately 1 standard sheet pan

~Variation: Slice bananas into coins for finger-size pieces.

Purple Tie-Dye Unicorn Muffins

This recipe is everything a professional pastry chef tries to avoid. But the kids adore the novelty of the purple muffin, so . . . go for it. My kids thought these muffins were absolutely magical. Although I don't usually advocate artificial ingredients, you can certainly find some naturally occurring gold shimmer dust online to top off the unicorn experience.

You'll Need

2 cups all-purpose flour
1 cup organic cane or coconut sugar
1/4 teaspoon kosher salt
3 teaspoons baking powder
1/2 extra virgin coconut oil, melted
2 eggs
1 cup milk or nut milk
1½ cups fresh blueberries, 1/2 cup smashed
Edible food-safe gold dust or gold leaf for the tops
Organic, nonstick cooking spray

Here's How

Preheat the oven to 375 °F. Line a muffin pan with cupcake papers, or prepare the muffin tin with your favorite organic nonstick cooking spray. Set aside. In a medium bowl, combine the flour, sugar, salt and baking powder.

In an additional bowl, combine the oil, the egg and the milk. Whisk to combine. Add the wet ingredients to the dry and combine. Fold in the 1/2 cup of smashed blueberries. Mix to color the batter purple without overbeating.

Gently fold in remaining berries. Fill muffin cups and bake for approximately 20 to 25 minutes until a toothpick inserted in the center of a muffin comes out clean.

Makes 12 muffins

~Variation: For traditional blueberry muffins, do not smash the blueberries; gently fold them into the batter.

Breakfast Nachos

I love, love, love, nachos for breakfast. And I love, love, love when I see my kids eating breakfast. This dish certainly ensures full bellies in the morning.

You'll Need

1 pound organic grass-fed hamburger meat

2 tablespoons organic butter

1 teaspoon fresh garlic, finely chopped

6 eggs, well beaten and seasoned with salt and pepper

1/4 teaspoon ground cayenne pepper

1/2 teaspoon garlic salt

1/2 teaspoon onion powder

1/2 teaspoon freshly ground black pepper

1/2 teaspoon paprika

1/4 teaspoon dry oregano

1/4 cup beef stock or water

1 teaspoon Worcestershire sauce

6 ounces restaurant-style tortilla chips

2 cups Monterey Jack cheese, shredded

1 medium tomato, deseeded, chopped

1/4 cup olives, sliced

Healthy, nonstick cooking spray

Sour cream (optional)

Salsa (optional)

Here's How

Heat the oven to 350 °F Spray a 13 x 9-inch baking dish with nonstick cooking spray; set aside. Salt and pepper the hamburger and cook in a 12-inch skillet over medium-high heat, stirring occasionally, about 5 to 8 minutes or until cooked through and crumbled; drain any excess fat.

Add the spices and dry oregano to the hamburger and stir to combine. Add stock and Worcestershire sauce; allow the hamburger to continue cooking through until almost dry, an additional 1 to 2 minutes.

Using a slotted spoon, transfer cooked hamburger to a small bowl. Cover and keep warm. Clean the skillet with a paper towel and return to low heat. Add the butter and heat until bubbly. Add garlic and sauté about a minute. Be sure not to brown— garlic inherently burns easily.

Add the seasoned, beaten eggs to the garlic butter, and continue to cook over low to medium heat, lifting egg mixture slightly with spatula to allow uncooked portion to flow underneath, about 3 to 4 minutes or until eggs are almost set. Then scramble.

While the eggs are cooking, spread half of the tortilla chips in a thin layer in the bottom of the prepared baking dish. Top the chips with half of the seasoned hamburger meat and 1 cup of cheese scattered over the seasoned meat. Repeat with remaining chips, hamburger, scrambled eggs, tomato chunks and cheese. Bake about 5 to 8 minutes or until cheese is melted; serve immediately, with sour cream and salsa if desired.

Makes approximately 6 to 8 servings

~An umami recipe

Breakfast Quesadillas

You'll Need

3 (10-inch) organic whole wheat or flour tortillas

3–4 teaspoons organic butter

1/2 cup green scallions, chopped (optional)

1/2 cup red bell pepper, diced small (optional)

6 large organic eggs, beaten

1 teaspoon Worcestershire sauce

6 slices turkey bacon, cooked and crumbled

6 slices of your child's favorite healthy cheese

Sour Cream Dipping Sauce (see recipe below)

1/2 ripe avocado, sliced

Here's How

Prepare the sour cream dipping sauce and set aside in the refrigerator to keep chilled. Spread about 1/2 to 1 teaspoon of butter on one side of each tortilla. Set aside.

Melt the remaining butter in a 12-inch nonstick skillet over medium-high heat. Add onions and bell peppers, cook about 2 to 3 minutes or until vegetables are tender. Add the beaten eggs, and continue cooking to a scramble. Remove and set aside; keep warm.

Wipe the skillet clean with a paper towel, and return it to the stove on low to medium heat. Place a tortilla in the pan, butter side down, and add a few tablespoons of the cooked egg mixture on one side of the tortilla. Top with cheese and bacon crumbles. Fold the other side of the tortilla over to form a half-moon shape. Press firmly with the back of a spatula, and cook until tortilla is browning and cheese is melted through. Flip and repeat until brown on the other side. Place the cooked quesadilla on a cutting board and cut into three triangles. Repeat with additional tortillas. Serve warm with sliced avocado and chilled sour cream dip.

Makes approximately 3 to 4 servings

~An umami recipe

Sour Cream Dipping Sauce

Kids either love cilantro or they really dislike it. If they prefer dip without it, simply remove it from the recipe.

You'll Need

8 ounces sour cream

2 tablespoons fresh cilantro, chopped

1 teaspoon fresh garlic, finely chopped

1/4–1/2 teaspoon ground cumin

Squeeze of lemon juice to taste

Sprinkle of garlic salt

Dash of soy or Worcestershire sauce

Here's How

In the sour cream container, combine all the ingredients and stir well. Reseal and place back into the refrigerator. Serve chilled.

Makes 1 cup

~An umami recipe

Green Monster Breakfast Muffins

Why not flex your parental power and establish a "green food" day of the week, introducing new green foods on that day? Call them whatever you want—these muffins are tasty.

You'll Need

4 cups raw baby spinach

3 overripe bananas

2½ cups all-purpose or gluten-free flour

1 teaspoon cinnamon

1/4 teaspoon allspice

2 teaspoons baking powder

1/2 teaspoon baking soda

1/2 teaspoon kosher salt

1 cup cane or coconut sugar

1½ cups butter

3 eggs

2 teaspoons vanilla

Here's How

Preheat the oven to in a preheated 350 °F. Spray two muffin tins with nonstick cooking spray and set aside. In the bowl of your food processor, combine spinach and bananas. Blend until spinach changes to a liquid state.

In a medium mixing bowl, combine the flour, cinnamon, baking powder, baking soda, salt and allspice. Mix well. Set aside.

In the bowl of your stand mixer or a large mixing bowl, add the sugar and butter. Mix on high speed until creamy and the sugar crystals begin to dissolve, about 2 to 3 minutes. Add eggs one at a time, mixing well in between each addition. Slowly beat in the spinach-banana mixture. Add vanilla.

Add the dry ingredients into the wet ingredients. Mix well to combine. Scoop the batter into the muffin tins. Bake for approximately 30 to 45 minutes or until muffins spring back to the touch and are slightly browned on edges. Test for doneness by running a toothpick in the center. If it pulls out clean, muffins are done.

Makes approximately 24 monster muffins

~Time-Saving Tip: Scoop the batter into the muffin tins using an ice cream scoop. This will assist with portion control and cause less mess.

Smoothies and Bowls

A smoothie is a blended, chilled, sometimes sweetened beverage made from fresh fruit or vegetables, and in special cases can contain chocolate. In addition to fruit, many smoothies include crushed ice, frozen fruit, honey, or sugar-free organic syrups. Often sipped through a straw or used in bowls and topped with delicious healthy fresh or dried fruits and nut toppings. Consumed any time of day. Pick up colorful straws and tiny drink umbrellas to have on hand when serving smoothies and mocktails!

Basics of a Fruit Smoothie

A smoothie's base is chopped fruit, either one type of fruit or several. When looking for the most nutritional value, berries are an excellent choice of fruit to use in a smoothie.

Blackberries, strawberries, raspberries and blueberries are packed with antioxidants and are excellent sources of fiber, vitamins such as B, C, and K, and minerals such as manganese, potassium and copper. Strawberries also contain omega-3 fatty acids. Anytime we can get these essentials into our little ones, we should, even if it means serving a smoothie for dessert or at any time of the day.

Textures

Many picky eaters have texture sensitivity. Ice and frozen fruits can act as smoothie thickeners. Low-fat Greek yogurt, which is a great source of calcium and amino acids, can also be used to thicken a fruit smoothie. Use your child's favorite liquid to make sure your smoothie blends well. Fruit juices such as grape, cranberry, orange or pineapple are not only good sources of antioxidants but also count as servings of fruit—just be sure to use 100 percent juice varieties. Other liquids that can be used include low-fat, skim, almond or soy milk.

Super De Duper Master Smoothie Formula

You'll Need

1 part fruit
1 part liquid
2 parts thick base

Here's How

To make a fruit smoothie, use 1/4 cup fruit, 1/4 cup liquid, and 1/2 cup of thickener such as ice or healthy plain yogurt. These measurements are not set in stone. You can add more liquid to make the smoothie thinner in consistency or add more thickener for a milkshake-like smoothie. Once fruit, thickener, and liquid are chosen and measured, place all the ingredients in a blender and blend until smooth. Quick and easy!

For added nutrition, supplements are often added to smoothies. Some common supplements added to fruit smoothies are soy or whey protein powder, vitamin C powder, wheat germ, and ground flaxseed. Check with your child's doctor regarding any additions.

Smoothies are a great nutritional way to serve up a refreshing dessert as well as breakfast. And with this basic recipe, your child can be in control of what is in her own special recipe. Take notes and write the ingredients down as you prepare and taste together. The worst thing is to have your child love the smoothies and you have no idea how to make it again.

Purple Dragon Buddha Bowl

Whoever thinks you cannot eat a smoothie out of a bowl is crazy, in my opinion. Your kids will love this naturally fragrant and colorful Buddha bowl and enjoy eating it with a spoon. Allow them to add their own toppings, and your morning should be off to a great start.

You'll Need

2 Pitaya Plus Organic Dragon Fruit Smoothie Packs

1–1½ cups coconut water

1 cup cashew or sweetened almond milk

1/2 cup frozen mango

1 cup frozen strawberries

1 scoop Vega Organic Vanilla Plant Protein

1 cup baby spinach

2 teaspoons chia seeds

1–2 tablespoons organic agave (optional)

Toppings

1 teaspoon cocoa nibs (optional)

1 banana, sliced

1 handful cashews, toasted and crushed

Toasted coconut

Additional sliced strawberries or any additional fresh fruit your child loves

Here's How

Place all ingredients in a standing blender or food processor and process on medium-high until the smoothie has reached the desired consistency. Add more or less liquid depending on your thickening preference. Ladle into individual serving bowls, and let your kids top with their favorite toppings!

Makes approximately 4 servings

~Time-Saving Tip: Pitaya Plus Organic Dragon Fruit Smoothie Packs can be found at Whole Foods in the freezer section or Amazon grocery delivery.

Dark Chocolate Banana Blueberry Smoothie

Yum, what a pairing! Did you know that dark chocolate is good for you? Teach the kids early to eat 70 percent and above cocoa and steer clear of the sugary stuff. This will be an added benefit extending into their adult life.

The ancient Mayans and Aztecs used cocoa for many homeopathic purposes, including constipation and diarrhea. Recent studies have shown that chocolate may be beneficial in thwarting these two conditions in children. A study in *The Journal of Pediatrics* showed that the flavonoids in cocoa limit the release of fluids that cause diarrhea, a condition that may lead to dehydration, which is a serious health problem for small children.

You'll Need

1 banana, cut up and frozen

1/2 cup frozen blueberries

4 tablespoons dark chocolate cocoa powder, unsweetened

1/2 cup baby spinach leaves

1/4 cup maple syrup or honey

3 cups vanilla-sweetened almond milk

1/2 cup ice cubes

Here's How

Place all the ingredients into your standing blender. Blitz and serve in cups with straws. Serve ice cold.

Makes approximately 2 to 4 servings

~Time-Saving Tip: Freeze fresh fruit on a small sheet pan in a single layer; once fruit is frozen, pack individual portions in freezer-safe containers. This will ensure you are using the best quality frozen fruit, and your smoothie will stay colder longer with the addition of frozen ingredients.

~Variation: If using frozen fruit, omit the ice cubes.

Peanut Butter and Jelly Smoothie

You'll Need

> 1/2 cup plain Greek yogurt
>
> 1 cup almond milk
>
> 2 tablespoons creamy homemade peanut butter, or almond butter if you prefer
>
> 1 cup fresh frozen strawberries or raspberries
>
> 1/2 cup ice cubes

Here's How

Place all the ingredients in your standing blender and process until smooth, about 1 to 2 minutes. Serve immediately.

Makes approximately 2 to 3 servings

~*Time-Saving Tip: Freeze the yogurt in ice cube trays and freeze the fruit to obtain a colder, much thicker smoothie. This recipe will hold in a thermos for up to 4 hours.*

Chapter Fourteen

BATTLE SNACK TIME | SNACK RECIPES

A snack is a small portion of food, in contrast to a regular meal. Traditionally, snacks are prepared from ingredients commonly available in the home, often leftovers, or sandwiches made from cold cuts, or nuts, fruit, cut veggies, and dips.

Snacks are a great way to be a "no-pressure" food fight parent. I suggest leaving snacks available for older children to graze on while doing homework between larger mealtimes, but only for a specific time period. Think "break-time." However, I also encourage you to keep your toddler and preschooler on a meal schedule.

During preschool years, growth is slow compared to the first 24 months of life, though kids still need a balanced diet that includes whole grains, lean meat, beans, low-fat milk, fruits, and vegetables.

Every age group has picky eaters. Some may be willing to eat but only on their terms and only certain foods. Healthy and well-timed snacks can help fill in mealtime nutritional gaps. They also can keep kids from getting overly hungry and cranky. If your picky eater gets cranky, getting him to eat new and improved

153

foods will be next to impossible. As mentioned before, controlled grazing times teach kids to manage their hunger because they learn when to expect the next scheduled mealtime. Avoid letting kids pick throughout the day, which can dull internal hunger cues and make them more likely to overeat.

Make sure you stock healthy snacks in your refrigerator or pantry. Snack foods that are high in calories, fat, and added sugar should be kept to a minimum or completely diminished. This doesn't mean kids can never have these foods, but rather that these foods should be offered only once in a while. Stay prepared so snacking can stay healthy.

Allow kids to choose their own snacks from among two or three nutritious options. Stay in control. By offering them a choice within the food groups, you are offering them independence within your parameters—again, a closed-ended choice.

Serve skim or low-fat milk, almond milk, or water with snacks instead of sugary drinks and soda. Limit 100 percent juice to one serving per day.

Don't allow the kids to eat in front of the television—or try not to; it's easier said than done. Serve snacks and especially meals at the family dining table unless you are eating at a designated playtime table—such as during teddy bear tea—or you are on the road, out and about carrying a packed lunch.

Never leave home without a stocked cold food storage bag. This will keep foods palatable. If you packed a snack and kept it at safe temperatures and the kids never ate it, just put it back in the refrigerator at home, saving money and frustration.

Keep an eye on how your child's moods affect eating patterns. Preschoolers often confuse boredom or fatigue with hunger. If your child just ate and is complaining of hunger again, see if a change of scenery or some active play could do the trick. Offer water. Many times, when humans feel hungry, they are really just thirsty.

Don't forget to actually share snacks with your child; she will follow your lead and eventually get the message that you're serving something good.

Allow your child in the kitchen. Sometimes kids that help with the food preparation will taste what they create.

Puffy Pesto Pizza Rolls

You'll Need

  1 cup mozzarella cheese, shredded

  1/2 cup Parmesan cheese, finely grated

  1 cup basil pesto

  2 sheets ready rolled puff pastry, thawed

Here's How

Preheat oven to 400 °F. Line two sheet pans with parchment paper or silicone baking mats, and set them aside. On a clean work surface, lay each sheet of puff pastry flat, with the short side of the rectangle facing you.

Divide the basil pesto equally and spread onto each sheet of puff pastry, covering the whole surface except a 1-inch border along the side furthest away from you. Divide the cheeses and sprinkle evenly on top of the basil pesto.

Roll the pastry into a log, leaving the plain edge until last. Brush the plain edge lightly with water, and pinch to seal. Place the logs, seam side down, on a cutting surface, and slice the roll into ½-inch discs. Place each disc on the baking sheets, spiral side up. Bake for 20 minutes or until golden brown. Serve warm or save for an additional snack.

  Makes approximately 16 pieces

  ~An umami recipe

Schlott's Knots Pretzels

You'll Need

  2½ cups all-purpose flour

  1 teaspoon kosher salt

  1 teaspoon sugar

  2¼ teaspoons active dry yeast

  ¾–1 cup warm water, not to exceed 115 °F

Topping

  6 cups water in a small saucepan

  3 heaping tablespoons baking soda

  1 large egg yolk, beaten (for optional shine)

  3 tablespoons butter, melted

  Pretzel or kosher salt for topping (optional)

Here's How

Combine the lukewarm water and sugar in the bowl of a stand mixer, and sprinkle the yeast on top. Stir. Allow to stand for 5 minutes or until the mixture begins to foam.

Fasten the dough hook attachment securely in place. Add the flour and butter while using the dough hook attachment, and mix on low speed until well combined. Change to medium speed and knead until the dough looks smooth and pulls away from the side of the bowl, approximately 5 to 6 minutes.

Remove the dough from the bowl, clean the bowl and then oil it with a light coating of healthy cooking spray. Return the dough to the bowl, cover with plastic wrap and set in a warm place for approximately 30 to 60 minutes, or until the dough has doubled in size.

Preheat the oven to 475 °F. Line a baking pan with parchment paper and lightly spray with cooking spray or use a silicon baking mat. Set aside.

Bring the 6 cups of water and the baking soda to a rolling boil in saucepan until baking soda dissolves. Remove from heat and cool.

In the meantime, turn the dough out onto a clean work surface and divide into 8 equal pieces. Roll each piece of dough into a 24-inch rope. Make a "U-shape" with the rope. Holding the ends of the rope, crisscross them over each other and press onto the bottom of the U in order to form the shape of a pretzel. Example: Top right should cross over to bottom left; repeat with the other side, left to right.

Place onto the prepared baking sheet pan. When you're ready, gently lower 4 of the 8 pretzels into the boiling water one by one and boil for about 2 minutes, spooning water over the top to give them a nice salty bath. This will assist in flavor as well as browning.

With a slotted flat spatula, remove the pretzels from the bath water. Return to the baking sheet; brush the top of each pretzel with the beaten egg yolk and water mixture and sprinkle with the pretzel salt. Allow them to rest about 10 additional minutes.

Bake until golden brown in color, approximately 8 to 10 minutes. Transfer to a cooling rack on top of a parchment-lined baking sheet for at least 5 minutes; brush with melted butter and top with more salt before serving.

Makes approximately 8 pretzels

Doris Cook's English Muffin Pizza

You'll Need

1 English muffin, split open with a fork

1 teaspoon organic butter or optional pizza sauce

2 slices real cheese

Here's How

Preheat the oven or toaster oven to 350 °F. Line a sheet pan with parchment or a silicon baking mat. Split an English muffin and spread each side with butter or pizza sauce. Add ham or any other toppings your child loves. Top with cheese and pop it in the oven. It takes only 2 to 3 minutes to heat through until cheese is bubbling.

If you want to put them in a lunch box for later, they taste great even when they're cold. Because the cheese has been melted it will hold its shape better.

I sometimes purchase pancetta in precut tiny cubes. I cook it and store it in an airtight container to use whenever I am making these mini pizzas. Sprinkle the precooked pancetta on top of the cheese before you pop it in the oven. Cheese-only mini pizzas are also a delicious snack option.

Makes 2 English muffin pizzas

~An umami recipe

Parmesan Zucchini Fritters

You'll Need

1 pound zucchini (about 2 large)

1/2 onion, finely chopped

3 large eggs, beaten

1/2 teaspoon garlic powder

Kosher salt and freshly ground black pepper

1/2 cup Parmesan, freshly grated

3/4 cup all-purpose flour

1½ tablespoons extra virgin olive oil

Dipping Sauce

1 cup homemade marinara sauce

5 large basil leaves, finely chopped

1 clove garlic, finely minced

Here's How

On the large holes of a box grater, grate zucchini into a cheesecloth or clean dishtowel, and squeeze out as much liquid as possible. Set aside.

In a large bowl, combine the grated zucchini with onion, eggs, and garlic powder. Season with salt and pepper and stir to combine. Add the Parmesan and flour and stir until the mixture's consistency is similar to cookie dough.

In a large skillet over medium-high heat, heat olive oil. For each fritter, scoop a heaping spoonful of the batter, press down into the pan to flatten, and cook until golden, about 2 minutes per side. In a small bowl, combine marinara with basil. Heat or serve cold for dipping.

Makes approximately 1 dozen medium fritters

~An umami recipe

Potato Pancakes with Cucumber Yogurt Dipping Sauce

Kids love potatoes, and pancakes and cucumbers. The combination of the three will be a huge hit.

You'll Need

2 large russet potatoes, peeled and grated
1/2 cup yellow or white onion, grated
2 eggs, beaten
3/4 cup whole wheat flour
1/2 teaspoon salt
Oil for cooking
Applesauce, for garnish
Creamy Cucumber Yogurt Dipping Sauce
(see recipe on the right)

Here's How

On the large holes of a box grater, grate the potato and onion into a cheesecloth or clean dishtowel, squeezing out as much liquid as possible, or blitz in your food processor. Set aside.

In a medium bowl, add the eggs, salt and pepper, and the potato and onion mixture. Stir to combine. Add whole wheat flour and stir again until incorporated well.

Heat a medium nonstick pan with a small amount of healthy cooking oil. With a spoon, place a heaping spoonful of the mixture in the hot, oiled pan, pressing down to form a round disc. Cook on medium-low heat until the potato cake has browned. Carefully flip and cook the other side until brown and crispy, about 2 to 3 minutes each side. Remove from pan and drain on paper towels.

Makes approximately 2 dozen small fritters

~*Variation: Use your imagination and experiment with other vegetables. Try combining the potatoes with corn kernels, scallions, peas, or carrots. Just remember to compensate for any excess moisture.*

Creamy Cucumber
Yogurt Dipping Sauce

Here are two great food pairings. Kids love the refreshing flavor of cucumbers and the tart tang and creamy texture of Greek yogurt. Another great hit, and it includes a serving of veggies and dairy! Use this sauce on sandwiches or as dip for cut-up veggies.

You'll Need

1 English cucumber, peeled and deseeded

2–4 cloves garlic, cleaned

1/2–1 teaspoon fresh lemon juice

1 cup plain Greek yogurt

1/4 cup dill, chopped (optional)

Kosher salt and ground white pepper to taste

Here's How

Peel and deseed the cucumber with a spoon. Rough chop the cucumber and place in a food processor with the garlic and lemon juice. Pulse to a paste. Add the yogurt and dill and pulse again to combine. Season with salt and pepper, serve chilled.

Makes approximately 1½ to 2 cups

~Refrigerate up to 1 week.

Whole Wheat Handheld Pot Pies

High in fiber, made with whole wheat white flour, and loaded with their own hearty meal, these are great for those days on the go. This recipe can be made in stages, a day ahead, or all at once. Kids love holding these in their own little hands.

You'll Need

Dough

>   1 large egg
>
>   3 cups whole wheat flour, plus more for work surface
>
>   1 tablespoons unsalted butter, cubed
>
>   3 tablespoons Parmesan cheese
>
>   1 tablespoon apple cider vinegar
>
>   1/4 teaspoon Kosher salt

Filling

>   2 tablespoons olive oil
>
>   1/2 medium onion, chopped
>
>   1 stalk celery, chopped
>
>   1 teaspoon fresh thyme, chopped
>
>   Kosher salt and freshly ground black pepper
>
>   4 tablespoons whole wheat flour
>
>   2 cups chicken broth
>
>   1 cup frozen peas and carrots, thawed
>
>   1/3 cup reduced-fat sour cream
>
>   1 cup rotisserie chicken, shredded, skin and bones discarded
>
>   1/4 cup fresh parsley leaves, loosely-packed, finely chopped
>
>   1 large egg, lightly beaten, for egg wash

Here's How

For the dough: Beat the egg with 3 tablespoons cold water in a small bowl. Set aside. Pulse the flour, 1/3 of the butter, and the Parmesan, vinegar, salt and pepper in a food processor until the mixture looks like fine bread crumbs. Add the remaining butter and pulse until the mixture is in pea-size pieces. Add the egg and pulse until the dough begins to come together. Turn the dough out onto a lightly floured, clean work surface. Divide the dough in half. Place each half on a sheet of plastic wrap and flatten into a disk. Set aside in the refrigerator to rest, minimum 1 hour. While the dough is resting, prepare the filling.

For the filling: Add the oil to a 4-quart high-sided saucepan over medium-high heat. Add the onion, celery and fresh thyme. Cook, stirring, until soft, about 5 minutes. Add the salt and a few grinds of pepper, stirring about 4 to 5 additional minutes.

Add the flour and cook, stirring, 2 minutes. Add the broth, peas, carrots and sour cream. Bring up to a boil, and then quickly reduce the heat to medium-low. Simmer until sauce reduces and starts to thicken, about 2 to 4 minutes. Stir in the cooked rotisserie chicken and parsley; adjust seasoning with salt and pepper to taste. Allow the mixture to cool completely. Set aside or store airtight until used.

To assemble: Preheat the oven to 375 °F. Line two baking sheets with parchment or nonstick silicone baking mats. Roll disk of dough on a slightly floured surface to about 1/8-inch thick. Using a 5-inch round cookie cutter, cut as many even numbers of rounds as you can. Gather the scraps, re-roll, and cut out remaining rounds. Repeat with the remaining disk of dough for a total of 24 rounds for both the top and bottom pieces of your 12 hand pies. If the dough gets too warm while you're working with it, wrap it back up in plastic wrap and chill it for about 15 to 20 minutes.

After all the dough has been cut into circles, place 12 dough rounds onto the prepared baking sheet. Brush the entire dough disc with egg wash. Place a few tablespoons of chicken pie filling in the center, carefully to not overfill. Top with another round and press with a fork on the outer edge to seal. Slit the top with a sharp knife to create a steam vent, and brush with additional egg wash. Bake the hand pies until they're golden brown and the filling begins to bubble, 15 to 18 minutes. Allow to cool significantly before serving.

Makes about 12 hand pies

~An umami recipe

~Time-Saving Tip: This filling can also be made a day ahead. Alternatively, freeze the unbaked pies for up to 1 month, then bake, from frozen, at 375 °F until they're golden brown, 20 to 24 minutes. Filling can also be made up to 1 month in advance and frozen in an airtight container.

Mini Square Cheddar Cheese Crackers

Count the ingredient list on this recipe below, compare it to one on the commercial brand crackers in your local grocery store, and then decide which one you would rather feed your family!

You'll Need

6 ounces sharp cheddar cheese, cubed small

1/4 cup salted butter, cut into pieces and softened

3/4 cup flour, sifted

1/2 teaspoon kosher salt

1/2 teaspoon ground white pepper

1 tablespoon whole milk

Here's How

Preheat oven to 350 °F. Line two baking sheets with parchment and a light layer of nonstick cooking spray or silicon baking mats, and set aside. Place first 5 ingredients in food processor and pulse until mixture turns into coarse crumbs. Add the milk and process until dough forms. Using your hands, form dough into a ball. On a clean, lightly floured work surface, flatten into a 1/8-inch disc. Cover airtight and chill for 30 minutes.

Remove from cooler and roll the best you can into a square shape. Using a pizza or pastry cutter, cut dough into 1-inch squares. Work quickly while the dough is cold, and it will hold its shape. Use the flat end of a wooden skewer to poke a hole in the center of each cracker. With a wide, flat spatula, transfer the cold dough squares to the prepared baking sheet at least a 1/4 inch apart.

Bake for 12 to 15 minutes, until edges start to brown. Do not overcook. Allow crackers to cool completely. Store in airtight container for up to 3 days in a cool place.

Makes approximately 4 to 5 dozen crackers

~Time-Saving Tip: Use a clean plastic kitchen ruler as a guide for your pizza cutter. This technique will give you an advantage by keeping your edges straight for a more uniform cracker.

~Variation: Add a sprinkle of Parmesan cheese to the top during the last few minutes of baking to create a rich umami flavor profile.

Roasted Chickpea Snacks

Falafel is a classic Middle Eastern dish of fried chickpea balls that are usually served in pita bread. This recipe uses the delicious flavors of falafel to make an easy, crunchy snack. Make only a batch at a time because they're really best when fresh.

You'll Need

2 (15-ounce) cans chickpeas, drained and rinsed with cold water

2 tablespoons good quality olive oil

2 teaspoons kosher salt

1 teaspoon ground cumin

1/2 teaspoon ground coriander

1/2 teaspoon garlic salt

Here's How

Preheat the oven to 350 °F. Prepare a cookie sheet with a nonstick cooking spray or a silicone-baking mat. Set aside.

Spread a layer of paper towels on the countertop, open the can of chickpeas, and drain excess water into the sink. Spread the drained chickpeas onto the paper towels and roll them around to remove any additional moisture. Set aside to air-dry while preparing the balance of the recipe.

Place the remaining ingredients into a small bowl and mix to combine. Add chickpeas and toss to coat. Place the coated chickpeas on the prepared baking sheet and spread evenly.

Bake until the chickpeas are crunchy and golden brown, about 1 hour, stirring halfway through to make sure they cook evenly. Remove the baking sheet from the oven and set it aside to cool for 5 minutes. Eat the chickpeas right away.

Makes approximately 2 cups

Broccoli Cheese Bombs

Meet the most delicious way your kids will eat broccoli, ever! Kids and adults love these little flavor bombs!

You'll Need

2 cups broccoli crowns, steamed

1 large egg

1/4 yellow onion

1/4 cup flat-leaf parsley, leaves only

1/2 cup cheddar cheese, grated

1 cup panko or Italian seasoned or gluten-free bread crumbs

2 cloves garlic

1/4 teaspoon garlic salt

1/4 teaspoon onion powder

Kosher salt and freshly ground black pepper

Pinch of ground cayenne pepper

Here's How

In the bowl of your food processor, combine the broccoli, onion, parsley and garlic. Pulse the broccoli mixture very fine, like rice.

In a medium bowl or gallon-size food storage bag, add the processed broccoli mixture with all of the remaining ingredients. Mix well with gloved or slightly wet hands to combine like you would make a meatloaf or meatballs.

Scoop mixture into the palm of your slightly wet hand. Roll the mixture into a ball. Once a ball has formed, begin pressing down on the top and bottom of the ball with your thumbs while pressing in on the sides with your other hand, rotating into a cylindrical "tot" shape.

Semi-freeze on a sheet tray, single file, for about 20 to 30 minutes—this will help to hold their shape while baking.

Preheat the oven to 400 °F. Remove the broccoli cheese bombs from the freezer and place onto your prepared baking sheets. Hit the tops with a spritz of healthy cooking spray and a dusting of salt and pepper.

Bake for 10 to 18 minutes. Turn the tots and bake an additional 5 minutes, or until golden brown.

Makes approximately 1½ to 2 dozen bombs

~*Time-Saving Tip: When shaping, leave the mixture in a ball shape and then flatten out into discs to save time. Will freeze airtight up to 1 month.*

Chapter Fifteen

BATTLE LUNCH

Lunch is a midday meal customarily served at noon or between two and four in the afternoon. In the UK and in parts of Canada and the United States, it is sometimes referred to as dinner; nonetheless, it is a midday meal. Feel free to give your picky eater the bulk of her nutritional requirements during this period, especially if she has played hard in the hours prior.

Lunch is a meal that varies in style more than breakfast. Toddlers and preschoolers could be at home with parents or caregivers, or they could be at daycare or preschool.

School-aged children can bring their own lunches to school or purchase lunch through their school lunch program. Luckily, the options for lunch are endless: anything from a complete home-cooked meal to creative sandwiches to sushi.

If all has gone well and your child has eaten breakfast and had a small snack midway between breakfast and lunch, she should be ready for something ample. Remember, particularly those of you with very young children, if you are using the "grazing techniques" discussed in the earlier chapters, offering a full sit-down lunch meal will be redundant if you're also offering snacks to your toddler during midmorning hours. She won't be hungry when she sits down to lunch and will be less likely to eat the foods that you want to offer her. Adjust accordingly. Use grazing techniques on days you will not require your child to also sit down to a full meal at lunchtime.

If your school-aged child is home for lunch, try to sit and eat together. Your child will be more likely to sit longer and might try new foods, especially if he has your attention and observes you eating the same foods you've offered him. Not to mention driving the children in the car or sitting at the table is when some of the best parenting opportunities are available to us. Take advantage of this time to connect with your child and enjoy light, positive conversations.

Making This Mealtime Stress Free

Lunch with Toddlers

Lunch with toddlers requires fortitude. The most important thing to remember with a young toddler is to not stress over the disorder, but don't be a pushover, either. Learn to teach, not punish.

Lunch with Preschoolers

When dealing with preschoolers or older toddlers, listen when they say they're not hungry. Try to remember their stomachs are only as big as their fists. Pick your battles; pushing a preschooler will only cause more resistance.

Lunch with School-Aged Children

Make sure your child wants what is in her lunch pack so she actually eats it and doesn't trade it, throw it out, or bring it home again. If a school-aged child is not able to select what's being packed, don't waste your time or your money. Give closed-ended choices and pack nutritious foods your child will actually eat, within reason. Leftovers are a great option for this age group.

The Brown Bag Alternative—Bento Boxes

Lunch does not have to continuously consist of a peanut butter and jelly sandwich with the crusts cut off and a side of veggie sticks. There are many other tasty and nutritious options, even for a brown-bag lunch. Get creative. Bento boxes are all the rage with school-aged kids. If you have time to pack a bento box, that is great. However, if you don't, spend some quality time with your school-aged children on bento box resources, and help them until they learn how to create one themselves and recognize the possibilities. Then you can count on them to help pack their own lunches.

Bento is the ancient Japanese tradition of packing lunch in a beautiful, decorative box, which contains small interior compartments, so portion sizes are easily controlled, and is usually filled with items from each food group.

Building a bento box for kids is an art and a great way to spend some creative, quality time with your child. For parents whose youngsters are thoroughly over sandwiches, join the trendy world of packing a bento-style lunch. Today, bento's stylish varieties contain carbohydrates, protein, fruits and veggies, and sometimes small treats. The foods are selected to provide a balance of colors, flavors and textures, and the process provides lots of fun for the producer as well as the recipient of the box.

The fun part of the bento is that it is meant to be cute, which delights little kids. Some people go all out when they're packing a bento box. They make exquisite food art that looks like cartoon characters and animals; however, this is not necessary. These lunches are really fun, but they're not something a realist parent is going to throw together early in the morning. We don't have masses of extra time to spend making our children's lunches into masterpieces.

Keep in mind you can build a bento after family dinner with leftovers, and you and your child can spend quality time doing it together. Who knows? You might decide to become an expert in bento building. Either way, enjoy your involvement.

When cooking in the kitchen with your child, remember

that it's the voyage, not the destination, that's important. Once your picky eater learns the novelty, she will want to get involved in the action. This is a great opportunity to use closed-ended choices when providing food options in this alternate lunch box.

If the bento box seems like a puzzle, that's because it is! View it in a noble way. This alternative lunchtime option can ensure that each food group is offered while your child is away from home.

The actual bento boxes come in a range of sizes. Choose one that holds about the same portion your child usually eats for lunch at home. You can select a slightly larger size so he can also eat his morning and afternoon snack out of the bento. For kids new to the alternative brown paper bag, familiarize lunch in the bento box a week before school starts; that way, your child will gain the experience of opening and closing the box as well as understanding the concept of packing. This is especially good for younger school-aged children. It will also give you a better sense of how much he'll eat, so you won't over pack.

Search the internet for an online store that showcases bento box accessories and ideas. Keep in mind that you will either love the bento box or develop animosity. Life as a bento box enthusiast could have you cursing my name or adoring me. You might become obsessed with your new hobby or dislike the extraordinary additional work you undertake as your addiction grows. Either way, just like anything else during our children's growth years, this too will pass; cuddle it while it's here. I hope you find excitement in these enchanting lunchtime ideas and embrace the joy the bento has to offer.

Bento Basics

You will need some sort of box to put your food in. Specialty shops and online stores sell dozens of different types of boxes designed specifically for bento meals. These boxes come in a variety of colors and shapes and range in price from about $2 for plastic boxes to much more for elaborate ones and fancy thermal lunch sets. Check Amazon to purchase bento boxes, detailed instructional books, and some fun equipment to help you design creative meals.

If you can find bento boxes, they're an easy way to go, but you can also use other types of containers without difficulty. Many commercial storage containers work just fine. You can find them at your local grocery market in the container and baking aisles. For a child's lunch box, I recommend a container that is close to 4 x 6 inches and about 1½ to 2 inches deep. This size will allow you to pack the box tightly and fill it up to the rim, which will keep the food from moving around and mixing together when it's in your child's backpack. One of the fastest, easiest ways to make the food in a lunch box look nice is to stack foods, line them up, or just generally give them some kind of order. There are many books and websites available for ideas on how to pack bento boxes for children.

Silicon Baking Cups

Most people use silicon baking cups to pack a bento. They are great for keeping moist foods away from dry and keeping small items like berries in one spot. They also add a splash of color to the bento presentation. You can use grease-resistant cupcake papers to start with.

Sharps

A regular kitchen paring knife will help. Use it for cutting sandwiches into strips, dicing fruit, cutting veggies into matchstick shapes, or cubing meats and cheeses. I might add that some people keep an X-Acto knife and sharp crafting scissors on hand specifically for bento activity.

Cookie Cutters

Invest in a few versatile cookie cutters to easily add a bit of "cute" to your lunches—a must-have for preparing bento lunches. Use smaller cutters in basic shapes like circles, stars or flowers, and a few larger cutters for sandwiches.

Sandwich Ideas

Waffles and Pancakes

Any child will look forward to feasting on a grilled cheese made with a savory or sweet waffle or pancake. Yep, thinking outside the box is the name of the bento box game! Turn lunch into brunch with a blueberry waffle sandwich with flavored cream-cheese filling, sugar-snap peas, cherry tomatoes, banana chips, and watermelon stars.

Pita Bread

The beauty of pita bread is that it is perfect for packing with your child's preferred fillings, and there is an assortment to choose from, including white, whole wheat, sesame, flax and so on.

Younger kids will be delighted to see a finger sandwich filled with something simple like butter, shredded cheese and lettuce, or ham or turkey. Older kids can try egg salad, cold cuts, tuna, and salmon, or just about anything else you can think of.

Flour Tortillas

Tortillas are multipurpose and available in various flavors and colors, including red tomato, green spinach and whole wheat. Spread a single tortilla with cream cheese, mayo, homemade ranch dressing, or mild goat cheeses, and then top with whatever you'd like.

Before rolling or folding, include washed and thoroughly dried lettuces, sprouts, olives, and baby spinach. Add sandwich meats, chicken or tuna salads, cheeses, or nut butters. Then roll it up and slice away!

Try introducing fun-shaped mini croissants, tiny bagels, square dinner rolls, soft Hawaiian sweet rolls, rice cakes, flat whole wheat lavash, or even whole grain hot dog buns. If your child prefers standard loaf bread, show her how to use cookie cutters to cut the sandwiches into amusing shapes. Young kids love the fun shapes children's bento boxes have a reputation for, so they might be beyond willing to try new fillings that they're usually wary of.

Pack a Variety of Foods

The whole idea surrounding children's bento boxes is to build a theme or variety of selections. If your child is not a sandwich eater, check out these alternate ideas.

Quesadillas

Spread refried beans on a whole wheat tortilla and sprinkle cheese on the top. Fold to make a half-moon. Heat a knob of butter in a sauté pan, about 1 teaspoon. Place the half-moon-shaped tortilla in the hot buttered pan and cook until brown, about 1 minute; flip and cook until the other side is brown, the beans are warmed through, and the cheese is melted. Slice into wedges, and you're all set to pack up! A cheese-only quesadilla is also an appealing option.

Hardboiled Eggs

If your child is eating at home, leave the shell on the egg so the child can peel it herself. Kids are more inclined to peel and eat eggs if the eggs are colored.

If your child is taking lunch to school, peel the egg before you pack it. This will make the protein-rich egg accessible to eat within the allowed lunch period. If she has to choose between allotting time to peel an egg or frolicking in the schoolyard, she might not eat the egg. You can purchase animal or flower-shaped egg molds at most bento supply stores online. This makes eating eggs beyond fun. They will show off.

Soups, Stews, or Chili

Most kids love soups, stews and chili. Not so much a bento option, but definably a school lunch option. These all work well for school-aged children. Just heat and pour into a thermos.

Boom, lunch is ready. Whichever the combination your child loves, pack it up! Chicken chili, tomato soup, vegetable stew, miso—the possibilities are endless. It's also a good idea to place the thermos in a large food storage bag just in case it opens in transport. Test the thermos and make sure the food is still warm after a few hours. Nothing worse than expecting a warm lunch and getting it at room temperature. A faulty thermos could create the perfect breeding environment for harmful foodborne bacteria. Bacteria grows after a two-hour holding window and thrives in temperatures between 40 and 140 °F. Keep hot foods hot and cold foods cold.

Sandwich Fillings

Use these on wholegrain breads, crackers, pita breads, rice cakes, flat bread, or just eat them on their own with a spoon. Other alternatives include avocado, grated carrots, sliced or diced cucumbers, flavored or plain cream cheeses, mild goat cheese, sprouts, cured salmon, tuna salad, sweet bell pepper rings, and egg salads.

Combine sliced leftover chicken with honey mustard, lettuce and tomato; try leftover grilled veggies with basil pesto and low-fat cheeses or cottage cheese alongside a stack of crackers; stick shrimp salad, dill and cucumber in a lettuce cup. Layer cheddar cheese with tart Granny Smith apple slices, bananas with fresh nut butters. Offer baked firm tofu, homemade popcorn with lunchmeats and grapes, chewy granola bars, or cookies with nut butters, just to name a few options. Avoid cucumber and tomato slices inside sandwiches; they can make the sandwich soggy, so pack them on the side.

One of the best thing about packing your child's lunch is tucking a note away for your child to find. For children that are not at reading age, draw a picture. My children looked forward to these little notes from home during their day, which prompted them to run to the lunch tables at mealtime. This can become a beautiful, positive family tradition that will be talked about for years to come.

Chapter Sixteen

LUNCH RECIPES

Turkey, Cheese, & Fruit Leather Rollups

Who says you need to make sandwich out of sandwich bread? Try this great pairing of fruit and cheese with the addition of turkey!

You'll Need

1 recipe fresh **Homemade Peach Fruit Leather**, or pear (see recipe below)

Sliced turkey breast

Whipped cream cheese

Kosher salt and freshly ground black pepper

Here's How

Unroll the fruit leather; spread the cream cheese the length of the fruit rollup except the last inch. Cut the turkey into strips that fit the width of the rollup and place on the cream cheese. Roll back up. Serve on its side.

Homemade Peach Fruit Leather

You'll Need

4 ripe peaches, pit removed, skin on, cut into chunks

1 teaspoon honey

Here's How

Preheat oven to 225 °F. Prepare the bottom of a sheet pan with parchment paper or a silicone nonstick baking mat, and set aside. Rinse and remove seeds from peaches. Place the peaches and honey in the bowl of your food processor or standing blender. Puree until smooth. Pour the mixture onto the prepared baking sheet and spread thin with a wet spatula to prevent sticking.

Bake for about 3 to 5 hours or until the edges look really dry and the center is not sticky to the touch. Baking times will vary depending on how thick you spread your mixture and how much juice is naturally contained in the fruit.

Set aside and cool to room temperature. Pull the dried fruit off the sheet pan onto your work surface, and cut in strips using clean kitchen scissors and leaving the parchment paper intact. Roll the leather up into cute bundles and secure with decorative kitchen twine. Keep airtight. These won't last long in your home.

Makes approximately 8 to 10 servings

~Variations: Replace the peaches with pears, plums or nectarines.

P B & J Sushi Rolls

As a chef, I believe kids should be in the kitchen as young as two to three years old with supervision. This recipe with nut butter and preserves will be a great introduction to getting kids involved in the kitchen.

You'll Need (per person)

2 tablespoons creamy nut butter

2 tablespoons of your favorite preserves

2 slices sandwich bread

Here's How

With a sharp knife, remove the crust from the bread. Using a rolling pin, completely flatten the bread while keeping the integrity of its shape. Spread the nut butter and preserves across the bread and carefully roll each slice into a tiny little spiral. Cut into four even pieces. Serve standing up to reveal the swirls of nut butter and jelly.

Makes approximately 2 servings

Cousin Rory's Cada Cada Toast

Psssst! Are you looking for a fast, cheap and easy snack? Me too! How about my cousin Rory's Cada Cada Toast—also known as avocado toast. Made with sprouted grain bread, which is very high in protein.

You'll Need

2 slices Ezekiel Whole Grain Sprouted Bread or your child's favorite bread

1 ripe succulent California avocado

Freshly ground black pepper

Garlic salt

Sliced veggies like red bell peppers, radishes, scallions

Here's How

Toast the bread to desired texture. Cut open the avocado and mash with a fork in a small bowl. Add the garlic salt and pepper to taste. Pile high on toast and top with sliced veggies. Gobble it up.

~*Time-Saving Tip: Because the loaf contains living sprouts, the bread will be found in the freezer section of your healthy grocery store. Sprouted grain bread contains things like legumes, millet, barley, oat, lentil and other grains that can provide a complete source of amino acids, the building blocks of proteins.*

Tasty Tropical Grilled Cheese Sandwich

You'll Need

2 slices whole wheat bread, each buttered on one side

2 slices of your child's favorite real cheese or soy substitute (non-processed)

1–2 slices good quality black forest ham, very thin, room temperature

1 pineapple ring, room temperature

2 tablespoons butter or organic spread, room temperature

Here's How

In a small sauté pan over medium-low heat, heat a teaspoon of the butter until bubbling; add pineapple ring and cook until caramelized and slightly brown, about 1 to 2 minutes on each side. Remove from the pan onto a paper towel. Set aside.

In the same pan, add both pieces of bread, buttered-side down. Top each slice of bread with a layer of cheese and black forest ham, add the pineapple to one of the pieces, and top with the other piece of bread, buttered-side up. Cook until bread is toasted on each side, flipping carefully and insuring the cheese is melting—about 2 to 3 minutes each side. Remove from pan and cut into four wedges. Serve warm.

Makes 1 sandwich to share

~An umami recipe

~Time-Saving Tip: Cold foods that are brought to room temperature prior to cooking will cook quicker and much more evenly.

Turkey Pho Gà

This is a fun twist on Vietnamese chicken noodle soup. In Hanoi, Vietnam, you'll find everyone enjoying delicious pho any time of day, for breakfast, lunch or dinner. Pho to the Vietnamese is the equivalent of burgers to Americans but better! This recipe is a great way to use up leftover turkey.

You'll Need

1 pound cooked turkey, shredded (about 4 cups)

6 whole scallions

1 shallot, peeled, root trimmed, and cut in half

Thumb-size piece ginger, peeled and crushed

1 tablespoon kosher salt

3 quarts chicken stock

Dash of fish or soy sauce, for seasoning

1 pound dried rice vermicelli, cooked

1 bunch scallions, thinly sliced

1 bunch cilantro, chopped

1 bunch Thai basil sprigs

4 cups mung bean sprouts

4 limes, cut into wedges

4 jalapeños, destemmed and thinly sliced into rings (optional)

Garnishes

Here's How

In a large, heavy-bottomed stockpot on high heat, combine the whole scallions, shallot, ginger, garlic, chicken stock, and fish sauce. Bring to a simmer—but do not boil—for about 35 minutes. Taste and add additional fish sauce or salt to season.

Add turkey. Turn off heat and set aside. Discard the cooked scallions and ginger from this pot. Prepare the soup garnish, and arrange the basil, mung sprouts, lime wedges and jalapeño slices on a serving platter. Divide the prepared rice noodles evenly among warmed soup bowls. Top each bowl with about 1/2 to 3/4 cup of the shredded turkey, and then divide the chopped scallions and chopped cilantro evenly among the bowls.

Ladle the hot stock over the top, dividing it evenly. Serve immediately, accompanied with the platter of garnishes. Let kids experiment with flavors by topping their own soup.

Makes approximately 6 to 8 servings

~An umami recipe

~Time-Saving Tip: Also great for evening meal the whole family can enjoy—a cook once, eat twice recipe.

Cold Tortellini Salad

You'll Need

1 pound fresh cheese-filled tortellini

1 English cucumber, peeled and deseeded, diced small

1 handful mini pear-shaped tomatoes

1 small red bell pepper, deseeded and diced small (optional)

1 carrot, grated

1 cup black olives

Sprinkle of garlic salt

Freshly ground black pepper

1 teaspoon extra virgin olive oil

1/2–3/4 cup of your child's favorite salad dressing

Here's How

In a large stockpot, bring water to a boil. Add the tortellini and cook as indicated on the package. Drain and rinse with cold water until cool. Toss in the olive oil to coat the pasta; this will prevent it from sticking. Combine the pasta with the remaining ingredients, cover with plastic wrap, toss with your child's favorite salad dressing, and chill before serving.

Makes approximately 4 to 6 servings

Turkey and Cheese Pita with Pineapple Carrot Slaw

You'll Need

1 whole wheat pita

Cream cheese, plain or flavored

1–3 ounces roasted turkey, thinly sliced, torn in pieces

1 red lettuce leaf

1 tablespoon Italian salad dressing

Pineapple Carrot Slaw (see recipe below)

Here's How

Cut the pita in half, spread the inside of each pita half with flavored cream cheese, and set aside. In a small bowl, toss the red lettuce leaf and the roasted turkey with Italian dressing and then place them inside the pita halves. Top with carrot pineapple slaw, or serve on the side.

Makes 1 pita sandwich

Pineapple Carrot Slaw

Here's How

> 10 pounds carrots, peeled and grated
>
> 1/2 cup dried currants or your child's favorite dried fruit
>
> 1 cup pineapple bits, drained
>
> 1/2 cup vanilla Greek yogurt
>
> 1 tablespoon honey

Here's How

Soak the raisins, currants or dried fruit in warm water for 15 to 30 minutes if your child prefers to eat them with a softer texture. Drain and dry.

In a mixing bowl, combine the dried fruit, pineapple and carrots. In a separate bowl, mix together the yogurt and honey. Add to the carrot mixture; mix well, cover and refrigerate until well chilled.

Makes approximately 8 to 10 servings

Focaccia with Grapes and Rolled Turkey

You'll Need

1/2 recipe of **Pizzette, Calzone and Focaccia Dough** (see recipe below) or healthy store-bought dough

2 tablespoons extra virgin olive oil

Coarse sea salt

1 clove garlic, minced

1 shallot, cut into thin rounds

1 tablespoon fresh rosemary leaves

1/2 cup green or red seedless grapes, cut in half

12 (2-ounce) slices fresh roasted turkey breast

3 ounces whipped flavored cream cheese

Infused Oil (see recipe below)

Here's How

Preheat the oven to 400 °F. Prepare a baking sheet with a light coating of cooking spray. Set aside. Roll the pizza dough into a rectangle and place onto the baking sheet, forming the shape of the pan by pressing and pulling the dough. Rest the dough for a few minutes in between stretching if it is snapping back. Once in place, using a pastry brush, cover the top of the dough with olive oil or additional infused oil. Sprinkle the dough with coarse sea salt, garlic, shallots and rosemary. Spread the grapes over the top and push them down into the dough.

Bake the focaccia until golden brown, about 25 minutes. While the dough is in the oven, spread cream cheese on the turkey slices and roll up into logs; chill in airtight container until the focaccia bread is ready.

When the focaccia is cooled from the oven, drizzle the infused oil on top. This is also a great way to get healthy oils into your child's diet. Cut into 12 slices and serve with 2 turkey breast rollups, or cut the rolls into spirals.

Makes approximately 12 servings

Pizzette, Calzone and Focaccia Dough

You'll Need

   5½ cups all-purpose flour

   1½ teaspoon salt

   1 teaspoons sugar

   1 package or 1/4 ounce fast acting dry yeast

   1 cup lukewarm water, not to exceed 110 °F

   2 tablespoons extra virgin olive oil

   2–3 tablespoons dry or fresh herbs, finely chopped
   (optional)

Here's How

In a large mixing bowl, combine flour, yeast, dried herbs and
1½ teaspoons salt. With a wooden spoon, stir in water and 3
tablespoons olive oil; beat mixture vigorously for 5 minutes.

Cover bowl with a clean towel, set aside and allow the dough
to rise in a warm place, away from drafts, until doubled in size
(about 40 minutes).

Turn dough onto a floured surface and gently knead for 1
minute. Lightly oil two large baking sheets (I use baking stones).
Divide dough in half, placing one half on each baking sheet.

Press or roll out each to a 10-inch round. Cover rounds with
clean towels and let rise until doubled in size (about 30 minutes).

Use this dough for a variety of uses. Best baked at 400 °F.

Makes enough for approximately 2 large focaccia breads, 5
individual pizzas, 10 mini calzones, or 20 mini pizzettes.

   *~Variation: Add 4 teaspoons dried or fresh herbs of your
   choice to the dough for added flavor*

Infused Oil

I use infused healthy oils to top pizzas and sandwiches, in vinaigrettes, to cook with, and to add to tomato bruschetta or just about anything that needs oil. Healthy oils add flavor, and they are a great way to get your children to intake their healthy fats.

You'll Need

1 cup best quality extra virgin olive oil

2 cloves garlic, peeled and smashed

10 black peppercorns

1/4 teaspoon crushed red pepper (optional)

1 sprig fresh thyme, rosemary, or your favorite herbs

1/4 teaspoon kosher salt

Here's How

Place all ingredients in a saucepan and heat to a simmer; do not boil. Remove from heat, cool, and place in an airtight glass jar, squeeze bottle or cruet. Serve with crusty bread for dipping or drizzle on finished foods. Do not strain. Experiment and try different combinations of herbs and spices.

Makes approximately 1 cup

~Store up to 1 week room temperature, or 2 weeks refrigerated.

Spicy Nut Butter Noodles with Grilled Chicken

Kids seem to live solely by eating nut butter sandwiches. Because of this tunneled food vision, I've paired nut butters with other foods. Some children just devour the additional ingredients when coated in warm creamy almond or peanut butters. Give it a try.

You'll Need

1/2 pound your child's favorite whole wheat pasta

1/2–3/4 cup creamy peanut or creamy almond butter

1 cup chicken stock

2 teaspoons reduced-sodium soy sauce

1/2 teaspoon toasted sesame oil or chili paste (optional)

1/2 teaspoon honey

1 medium carrot, peeled with vegetable peeler into long ribbons

1 celery stalk, peeled and thinly sliced on an angle

1 cup broccoli, cut into bite-size pieces

2 chicken breasts, pounded thin

Here's How

Cook whole wheat pasta according to package directions. Season the chicken with salt and pepper, drizzle with a little oil and grill until done. Set aside and keep warm. While the pasta is cooking, warm the nut butter with the soy sauce, sesame oil, and honey in a small saucepan over low heat. Stir to combine, keep warm and set aside. When noodles are ready. Drain and place back into the pot they were cooked in, add the peanut sauce, and toss to coat well. Serve with the grilled chicken.

Makes approximately 4 to 6 servings

~An umami recipe

~Time-Saving Tip: Serve warm or cold.

Homemade Mayonnaise

If your child is a sandwich eater, why not make your own mayonnaise? Your family will then be eating a healthier version of the pantry staple, and not one burdened with trans fats or shelf stabilizers we cannot pronounce. There are a few ways to make mayonnaise. I use my food processor with the small bowl attachment, but an immersion blender or making it completely by hand will work; just make sure all your ingredients are at room temperature.

You'll Need

1 organic egg, room temperature

1 organic egg yolk

1 teaspoon Dijon mustard

1 teaspoon apple cider vinegar or fresh lemon juice

1 cup extra light neutral-flavored healthy oil

Kosher salt and paprika to taste

Here's How

Place 1 egg and the yolk of the other in your blender, along with the Dijon and cider vinegar or lemon juice. Process approximately 30 seconds or until frothy. Continue to run the food processor while slowly adding the oil in small droplets until about 1/4 of the oil has been added. Mayonnaise is a temperamental primary culinary sauce. By introducing the oil slowly, the mixture has less risk of separating.

Once 1/4 cup of the oil has been successfully added, you should notice the mixture beginning to thicken and emulsify. Once this happens, you can be a little less strict with how slowly the oil is added. A thin stream is perfect now, and you'll be left with thick and creamy mayonnaise. Add salt to taste. Transfer to a small, pint-size jar and close the lid tightly. Refrigerate.

Makes approximately 1 cup

~Time-Saving Tip: If your mayonnaise separates, don't worry. In an additional bowl, add about 1 teaspoon of mustard and then slowly beat the broken mayonnaise into the mustard until it becomes emulsified and creamy again. Another trick is to repeat the same process but replace the teaspoon of mustard with an additional egg yolk.

Chapter Seventeen

BATTLE DINNER |
DINNER RECIPES

At one time, dinner was the main meal of the day. However, depending on your culture, it may now be second, third, or fourth in terms of importance. This meal usually takes place at the end of the day, when most of us can gather around and relax and share time with other family members.

Statistics show that children in most families that share this mealtime are less likely to have drug and alcohol abuse problems, especially during the teen years.

Whether you're cooking a gourmet meal, ordering food from your favorite take-out place, or eating on the go, what your kids really want during dinnertime is *you*! Family meals are the perfect time to talk to your kids and to listen to what's on their minds.

Family Day™, a day to eat dinner with your children, is a national movement launched in 2001 by the National Center on Addiction and Substance Abuse to remind parents that frequent family dinners make a difference.[15] Substance abuse can strike

---

15   The National Survey of American Attitudes on Substance Abuse XIV: Teens and Parents from March 2 to April 5, 2009 (teens) and March 21 to April 10, 2009 (parents). The firm interviewed at home by telephone a national random sample of 1,000 12-to-17-year-olds (509 boys, 491 girls) and 452 of their parents. Sampling error is +/- 3.1% for teens and +/- 4.6% for parents.

any family regardless of ethnicity, affluence, age or gender. The parental engagement fostered at the dinner table can be a simple, effective tool to help prevent substance abuse in kids. Family Day began as a grassroots initiative and has grown to become a nationwide celebration; in 2009, President Obama, all the state governors, and more than a thousand mayors and county executives proclaimed and supported Family Day.

Oodles of Vegetable Noodles

Want to try something different? Buy a spiralizer and make your family oodles of noodles from zucchini, sweet potatoes, carrots or summer squash. You can readily purchase noodles made from zucchini, carrots, or sweet potato, but they will be dried out in the package, and likely the supplementary nutrition will be depleted. With a spiralizer machine, the kids will really want to get involved.

I use Paderno World Cuisine's 3-Blade Spiral Vegetable Slicer. This is the quickest tool on the market and requires the least amount of strength or effort, with suction cup feet to keep it in place, and it's under $30. You simply cut off the ends of a zucchini, carrot, sweet potato or beet and place it in the apparatus and spin. In less than 10 seconds, you'll have spiraled an entire vegetable.

Spiralizing is a great way to increase vegetables in your family's diet and an alternative to pasta that's gluten free, grain free, wheat free, low carb, healthy and nutritious, inexpensive, easy to prepare, unprocessed, and vegan.

Make your zoodles ahead of time! This the best time-saving tip. After you've spiralized several zucchini, line a large glass storage container with a paper towel; add your noodles and place in the refrigerator. They'll stay fresh for 2 to 3 days. Larger zucchini are easier to spiralize and will yield more noodles; plan on one medium zucchini per person.

To peel or not to peel the zucchini? I don't peel the zucchini before spiralizing, as I love the added green in my dish and extra nutrients it provides, like dietary fiber. Don't forget to make zucchini ribbons and spiralize lots of other veggies. Get creative.

When making zoodles from zucchini, I use white-fleshed zucchini because it is so beefy. I often combine white and green zucchini and throw in a yellow crookneck squash for color. I don't even cook them. Heat your sauce and toss the zoodles right in the pan. They will heat through without getting soggy. Watch out for the release of water for the zoodles and drain—zucchini are 95 percent moisture.

Zuccetti with Marinara Sauce

Zoodles are a fun, fresh and healthy alternative to pasta—certainly a way to increase the amount of vegetables you and your family eat. Zoodles are nutritious and a healthy alternative to highly processed foods.

You'll Need

1 tablespoon olive oil (optional) or 1 spray of good quality cooking oil

1 onion, peeled and roughly chopped

2 cloves garlic, cleaned and roughly chopped

1 tablespoon each fresh oregano, marjoram, rosemary and thyme leaves, chopped

Pinch of crushed red pepper (optional)

1/2 cup fresh flat-leaf Italian parsley

1/4–1/2 cup chicken or vegetable stock

2 (14-ounce) cans organic chopped tomatoes

Kosher salt and freshly ground black pepper (optional)

3–4 large zucchini, washed, dried and spiralized

Here's How

In a large, heavy-bottomed sauce pan set over medium heat, add the oil and heat for about 30 seconds. Add the onion and cook until translucent and starting to turn brown, about 1 to 2 minutes.

Add the garlic and the herbs. Sauté an additional 1 minute to release flavors. Deglaze the pan with the stock and remove any brown caramelized bits from the pan.

Add the tomatoes and crushed red pepper flakes. Reduce the heat to low. Simmer, uncovered, until the tomatoes soften, and sauce is reduced by 1/3, about 15 minutes.

Adjust seasoning with salt and fresh ground pepper. Remove from heat and liquefy to a sauce with your immersion blender, food processor or blender. Serve on top of fresh prepared raw room temperature zoodles or cool and store airtight for a later date.

Makes approximately 4 servings

~*Special Equipment Needed: A spiralizer*

Zoodles with Lemony Garlic Shrimp

You'll Need

2–3 teaspoons olive oil or extra virgin coconut oil

1/2 medium yellow onion, cleaned and julienne-sliced

1/2–1 cup grape tomatoes, halved

1 teaspoon crushed red pepper

4 cloves garlic, cleaned, cut and smashed to paste

Himalayan salt and freshly ground black pepper to taste

1 pound fresh shrimp (30–32 size), peeled and deveined

Juice and zest of 1 lemon

1/4 cup fresh Italian parsley, finely chopped

1/4–1/2 cup chicken or vegetable stock to deglaze

4–6 medium zucchini, spiralized

Here's How

In a medium nonstick skillet, heat oil over medium-high heat. Add the onion and sauté until almost translucent, about 1 minute. Add the tomatoes, garlic and 1 teaspoon of crushed red pepper flakes if using. Sauté for an additional minute. Season the shrimp with salt and pepper and add to the pan. Cook 2 to 3 minutes until shrimp begin to turn pink.

Add the lemon juice and continue to cook 1 to 2 additional minutes until the shrimp are just cooked through and opaque. Do not overcook. Deglaze the pan with stock; allow to reduce about 2 minutes to make a quick, flavorful pan sauce. Taste and adjust seasoning with salt and pepper. Pour over gently warmed noodles, toss and serve immediately.

Makes approximately 4 to 6 servings

Zucchini and Kale

You'll Need

6 white-fleshed or green medium zucchini, spiralized into zoodles

10 leaves fresh curly kale, stems removed

1/4 cup fresh roasted almonds

2 cloves garlic, cleaned

1/4 to 1/2 teaspoon garlic salt

1 tablespoon extra virgin olive oil or extra virgin coconut oil, melted

1 tablespoon Parmesan cheese, freshly grated

1 bunch large basil leaves

Kosher salt and freshly ground black pepper to taste

Ice

Here's How

Fill a small stockpot with water and bring to a rapid boil. While waiting for water to boil, set a mixing bowl in the sink with a few cups of ice. Fill with cold water and leave inside the sink.

After removing the thick central stalk from the kale leaves, plunge the kale into the boiling water. Boil the leaves for about 1 minute, quickly remove from the water, and plunge into the cold water to stop the cooking process. Remove from the ice bath and drain on paper towels. Blot away any additional moisture.

In a food processor, add the blanched kale, garlic, nuts, Parmesan cheese and basil leaves. Pulse until close to liquefied. Add the extra virgin olive oil in a drizzle through the feed tube while the processor is on to create an emulsion. Taste and adjust seasoning with salt and pepper. Heat the kale basil pesto and toss through room-temperature zoodles. Serve immediately.

Mini Taco Salads in Tortilla Cups

Kids love tacos. I love anything mini and in a cup. Muffin tin cookery makes portion control easy and also makes for handy grab-and-go compact meals.

You'll Need

12 (6-inch) flour tortillas

2 tablespoons vegetable oil, separated

1 pound lean ground beef or ground turkey

1 onion, diced small

2 cloves garlic, minced

1/2 cup crushed canned tomatoes, drained

1/2 cup beef stock

1 teaspoon chili powder

1 teaspoon ground cumin

1 teaspoon dried oregano

1/2 teaspoon garlic salt

Filling

1/2 head iceberg lettuce, thinly sliced

1 cup cheddar cheese, shredded

1 avocado, diced

1 cup black beans, drained and rinsed

1 cup sliced black olives, drained

12 cherry tomatoes, quartered

1/2 cup of your favorite salsa

Here's How

Preheat the oven to 425 °F. Spray a muffin tin with cooking spray and set aside. Cut the tortillas with a 4-inch cookie cutter ring and cover with a damp paper towel; heat the tortillas in the microwave for about a minute to make pliable.

Dipping your fingers in oil, rub both sides of the tortilla lightly. Place the slightly oiled flour tortilla into the muffin cup and press down so it adheres to the bottom of the cup; pay special attention to ensure the sides of the tortillas are not collapsing in. If a few of the tortillas refuse to stand up, make a loose ball of foil and place inside the tortilla to keep from collapsing during baking.

Bake until golden brown, about 10 to 12 minutes. Cool completely. Gently remove from muffin tin to make sure they are not stuck. Replace, and fill the baked tortillas with prepared filling, top with cheese, and return to the oven for about 2 to 3 minutes to melt cheese in the oven and heat the toppings.

Makes 12 taco cups

~Time-Saving Tip: Store airtight if making ahead.

Lemon Parmesan Chicken Cutlets

You'll Need

3/4 cup all-purpose flour

2 large eggs

1½ cups panko

1/4 cup Parmesan, grated

1 tablespoon mustard powder

Kosher salt and freshly ground pepper

4 small skinless, boneless chicken cutlets (about 1½ pounds total), pounded to 1/4-inch thickness

8 tablespoons olive oil, divided

1 lemon, halved

Here's How

Place flour in a shallow bowl. Beat eggs in a second shallow bowl. Combine panko, Parmesan, and mustard powder in a third shallow bowl and season mixture with salt and pepper.

Season chicken with salt and pepper, then dredge in flour, shaking off any excess. Transfer to bowl with beaten egg and turn to coat. Lift from bowl, allowing excess to drip back into bowl.

Coat with panko mixture and press to adhere.

Heat 6 tablespoons oil in a large, heavy skillet or a cast-iron skillet over medium-high heat. Working in 2 batches, cook cutlets, adding remaining 2 tablespoons oil to the pan between batches, until golden brown and cooked through, about 4 minutes per side. Transfer cutlets to a paper-towel-lined plate and season with salt. Serve with fresh lemon wedges.

Makes approximately 4 servings

~Time-Saving Tip: Chicken can be breaded 3 months in advance. Place on a flat sheet pan between pieces of freezer paper or waxed paper and freeze. Once frozen individually, gather and place together in one airtight lined container and pull from the freezer as needed. Thaw before cooking.

Chicken Parmesan Casserole

You'll Need

2 pounds boneless, skinless chicken breasts

½ cup all-purpose flour

3 large eggs

2–3 cups panko, as needed

Kosher salt, as needed

Freshly ground black pepper, as needed

Olive oil, for frying

5 cups **Smooth Sweet Basil Marinara Sauce** (see recipe below)

1 cup Parmesan, preferably Parmigiano-Reggiano, finely grated

½ pound fresh mozzarella, torn into bite-size pieces

Here's How

Heat oven to 400 °F. Prepare a 9 x 13 baking dish with a spritz of nonstick cooking spray. Set aside.

Place the chicken between two pieces of parchment paper, wax paper, or inside a gallon food storage bag. Using a kitchen mallet or rolling pin, pound meat to even, 1/4-inch-thick slices.

Add flour, eggs, and panko respectively to three individual, shallow containers. Season the pounded chicken generously with salt and pepper on both sides. Dip a piece in the flour, then into the eggs, and then press into the panko mixture. Repeat until all the meat is coated.

Fill a large skillet with a 1/2-inch of oil. Place over medium-high heat. When oil is hot, fry cutlet in batches, turning halfway through, until golden brown. Transfer to a paper-towel-lined plate.

Spoon a thin layer of the tomato sauce over the bottom of the baking dish, then sprinkle one-third of the Parmesan over sauce. Place half of the cutlets over the Parmesan and top with half the mozzarella pieces. Top with half the remaining sauce, sprinkle with another third of the Parmesan, and repeat layering, ending with a final layer of sauce and Parmesan.

Transfer the baking dish to oven and bake until cheese is golden and casserole is bubbling, about 20 minutes. Allow to cool a few minutes before serving.

Makes approximately 6 to 8 servings

~An umami recipe

~Variation: Place a thin slice of prosciutto over each cutlet before adding sauce and cheese.

~Time-Saving Tip: Chicken can be breaded 3 months in advance. Place on a flat sheet pan between pieces of freezer paper or waxed paper and freeze. Once frozen individually, gather and place together in one airtight lined container and pull from the freezer as needed. Thaw before cooking.

Smooth Sweet Basil Marinara Sauce

Red sauce in less than 30 minutes. Most picky eaters will not eat tomato-looking chunks; this is a great recipe for those kids.

You'll Need

4 tablespoons extra virgin olive oil

3 tablespoons butter

1 large yellow onion, finely diced

3 large cloves garlic, minced

5 cups canned tomato chunks

1 cup vegetable or chicken stock

1 teaspoon kosher salt

Freshly ground black pepper

1 bunch fresh parsley, chopped

1/4 cup fresh marjoram, chopped

1/4 cup fresh thyme leaves

10 large basil leaves, chopped last minute

Here's How

Heat the olive oil in a medium-large stockpot over moderate heat. Add the onions and garlic and sauté until brown and caramelized, about 5 minutes. Add the stock and tomato puree and bring to a simmer. Add the parsley, half the basil, all of the marjoram, and all of the thyme leaves.

Simmer until reduced to a sauce-like consistency, about 15 minutes. Taste and adjust the seasoning if necessary. If the sauce tastes too acidic, add more stock and cook for 15 more minutes. If it needs a touch of sweetness, add sugar or honey to taste. Cook for 10 to 20 more minutes, reducing liquid by 1/4 if you have time.

Submerge your immersion hand blender into the sauce, and puree until smooth. Adjust seasoning with salt and pepper.

Reduce liquid again by an additional 1/4 if you have time. Chop the remaining basil and add to sauce.

    Makes over 1 quart of sauce

    ~An umami recipe

    ~Time-Saving Tip: Can be made up to a month in advance and frozen until use. Use for pizza, empanadas, or stromboli recipes.

Chicken Enchilada Casserole

I don't know about you, but I never have time to properly roll up individual enchiladas. I thought it would be much more logical and time saving to layer the ingredients to make a casserole instead. Sometimes we need to think about the whole family, and when we have a picky eater it's nice to be able to present a dish that is diverse but still contains recognizable flavors of beloved comfort foods.

You'll Need

1 cup rice

4 tablespoons olive oil

4 large beefsteak tomatoes, diced small

2–3 cloves garlic, minced

1 large onion, diced small

1/4 teaspoon chili powder

1 teaspoon paprika

1 teaspoon ground cumin

1/4 teaspoon ground white pepper

1 rotisserie chicken, skin removed and meat torn into bite-size pieces

Kosher salt and freshly ground black pepper

2 cups chicken stock

1 (15-ounce) can black or pinto beans, drained and rinsed

1 (15-ounce) can kidney beans, drained and rinsed

1 (16-ounce) container of your favorite fresh salsa

15–20 (8–10-inch) fresh corn tortillas

1 (11-ounce) can of corn, drained

1½ pounds cheddar cheese, grated

1 (16-ounce) can red enchilada sauce

Sour cream, for garnish

Fresh cilantro, chopped, for garnish

Here's How

Preheat the oven to 375 °F. Cook the rice according to the package directions. Set aside. Prepare a 9 x 13 ovenproof casserole dish with nonstick cooking spray. Set aside.

In a large skillet over medium-high heat, warm 2 tablespoons of the oil and add the tomatoes, garlic and onions. Stir and cook until onions are transparent. Add the chicken with the chili powder, paprika, cumin and some salt and pepper. Mix to coat chicken well and toast the spices about 2 to 3 minutes. Add 1 cup chicken stock and stir to make a sauce. Allow the sauce to boil until reduced by half, about 5 minutes.

Stir in the pinto and kidney beans and set aside. To assemble, place about a cup of salsa in the bottom of the 9 x 13 dish. Layer half of the tortillas on top of the salsa, overlapping the edges. Spoon the rice over the tortillas and spread until covered. Now layer the tomato mixture over the rice and sprinkle the corn over the tomatoes. Next, add the chicken and bean mixture, and then sprinkle on half the cheese and pour half the enchilada sauce. Continue with the same sequence of layers, finishing with the layers of tortilla on top. Cover in enchilada sauce and top with cheddar cheese.

Cover the casserole with aluminum foil and bake for 20 minutes. Remove the foil and continue baking until hot and bubbly, 15 to 20 minutes. Allow the casserole to sit for a few minutes before serving.

Serve with sour cream and cilantro for topping. Tastes even better the next day.

Makes approximately 12 servings

~An umami recipe

Auntie Allie's Tamale Pie

Tamale pie is an old-school comfort food and was developed sometime in the early 1900s. Some dispute this historic casserole type meal could have originated in Texas. It's first known published recipe dates way back to 1911. My family loved this dish, and my aunt Allie was famous in our family for her recipe.

You'll Need

2 teaspoons good quality olive oil

1 onion, diced small

3 cloves fresh garlic, cleaned and finely diced

1 (4-ounce) can diced green chilies, drained

3–4 cups cooked chicken or leftover turkey meat, shredded

1 tablespoon ground chili powder

1 tablespoon ground cumin

1 teaspoon ground oregano

1 teaspoon garlic salt

1 lime, juiced

1 cup of your favorite fresh or prepared salsa

2 cups of your favorite enchilada sauce

1 (12-ounce) can black beans, drained and rinsed

1 cup corn kernels

1 cup sliced black olives

1½–2 cups chicken broth

4 scallions, sliced

1 cup cornmeal

1 cup cheddar cheese, grated medium

1 tablespoon unsalted butter

Kosher salt and freshly ground black pepper

Garnishes

Sour cream

Black olives, sliced

1 bunch cilantro, chopped

2 beefsteak tomatoes, chopped

1 serrano chili, sliced, deseeded and veins removed
for less heat

Mexican cheese, crumbled

Here's How

Prepare a 13 x 9 ovenproof baking dish or a large cast-iron pan with nonstick cooking spray and set aside. If using the cast-iron pan, prepare everything on the stove and transfer to the oven, bypassing the baking dish. If not, use a large, high-sided saucepan over medium heat and warm the turkey with the salsa, enchilada sauce, beans, onions, 1/2 cup stock, chili powder and cumin. Stir to combine and bring to a simmer; allow the flavors to combine about 8 minutes. Remove from the heat and gently fold in the scallions and sliced black olives. Set aside.

In a medium saucepan, combine the cornmeal with the remaining 2 cups of chicken broth. Bring to a simmer over medium heat, stirring, until very thick, 5 to 7 minutes. Remove from the heat, and stir in the cheddar cheese and the butter. Taste and adjust seasoning with salt and pepper.

Spread the cornmeal mixture over the filling and bake at 400 °F until cooked through, about 20 to 30 minutes. Let stand for 10 minutes after you remove the dish from the oven. Serve warm with a platter full of delicious garnishes.

Makes approximately 12 to 14 servings

~An umami recipe

Blueberry Pancake Casserole

Why not make breakfast for dinner? This recipe is great because the kids will love that you're serving it for a family meal, and you can serve the leftovers for breakfast! This recipe is sure to be a win-win!

You'll Need

Pancakes

- 1¾ cups all-purpose flour
- 1½ teaspoons baking powder
- 1 teaspoon baking soda
- 1 teaspoon table salt
- 2 teaspoons granulated sugar
- 2 cups buttermilk
- 2 large eggs
- 1/4 cup salted butter, melted
- 1 pint blueberries, washed and dried
- Butter, for greasing griddle or pan

Casserole

- 1½ cups heavy cream
- 1 cup whole milk
- 6 large eggs
- 1 teaspoon vanilla extract
- 1/4 teaspoon ground cinnamon
- 1/4 cup granulated sugar
- 3/4 cup fresh blueberries
- 1 cup pure maple syrup
- 2 tablespoons butter, melted

Here's How

For the pancakes: In a large bowl, stir together the flour, baking powder, baking soda, salt, and 2 teaspoons sugar; make a well in the center and set aside.

In an additional bowl, whisk together the buttermilk and 2 eggs. Slowly stir into flour mixture. Gently stir in 1/4 cup melted butter and fold in blueberries. Batter will be lumpy. Allow to rest for 5 minutes.

Heat a large nonstick griddle over medium-high. When hot, lightly coat with butter. Drop 1/4 cup batter per pancake with a ladle, and make a circular motion with the back of the ladle to form the batter in a circle on the griddle; cook until tops of the pancakes are full of bubbles, about 3 to 4 minutes.

Flip and cook until golden brown, 3 to 4 minutes. Repeat with remaining batter to make about 20 pancakes.

To assemble: Cut each pancake in half. Set aside. Prepare an 11 x 7-inch baking dish with cooking spray. Stand pancake halves, cut-side down, in 2 rows; start at the short end of the prepared baking dish and fill the dish completely, slightly overlapping pancake edges down the center of the dish. Set aside.

Whisk together cream, milk, eggs, vanilla, cinnamon, and 1/4 cup sugar in a large bowl. Slowly pour mixture over pancakes. Cover and refrigerate at least 8 hours or overnight.

Preheat oven to 350 °F. Uncover casserole; top evenly with blueberries. Bake in preheated oven until center is set, 50 to 55 minutes. Let stand 5 minutes.

Heat maple syrup and butter in a small pan over low heat until heated through and butter is melted. Drizzle 1/4 cup syrup mixture over casserole and serve remaining syrup on the side.

Makes approximately 8 to 10 servings

Lasagna Cups in Wonton Wrappers

Easiest lasagna you'll ever prepare. Conveniently made into single servings that taste great warm or cold. This is a great quick homecooked food, great for those on-the-go mealtimes, and a great addition to bento boxes.

You'll Need

  1 tablespoon olive oil

  2 Italian sausage links, casing removed

  1 cup marinara sauce, homemade or your favorite Bolognese

  1½ cups ricotta cheese

  Kosher salt and freshly ground black pepper to taste

  24 (2-inch) wonton wrappers

  1½ cups mozzarella cheese, shredded

  1/2 cup Parmesan cheese, finely grated

  2 tablespoons fresh parsley leaves, chopped

Here's How

Preheat oven to 375 °F. Lightly spray a 12-cup standard muffin tin with your favorite nonstick cooking spray and set aside.

Heat olive oil in a large stockpot over medium heat. Add Italian sausage and cook until browned, about 3 to 5 minutes, making sure to crumble the sausage as it cooks and drain excess fat, and stir in marinara sauce. Season ricotta cheese with salt and pepper to taste; set aside. Fit wonton wrappers into each of the 12 muffin tins, pressing carefully to make sure there is an opening in the center.

Fill each cup with 1 tablespoon ricotta cheese at the bottom. Top with 1 tablespoon marinara and sausage combination, 1 tablespoon mozzarella cheese, and a sprinkling of grated Parmesan. Repeat with an additional layer. Top with Parmesan.

Place the muffin tin on a baking sheet and bake for

approximately 10 to 12 minutes, or until the cheese has melted and the wonton wrappers are golden brown.

Makes 12 servings

~*An umami recipe*

~*Time-Saving Tip: Prepare the entire ingredient list ahead of time, up to 3 days in advance. Assemble as needed. Do not freeze.*

Southwestern Egg Rolls

You'll Need

1 cup organic canola oil, for frying

24 (2-inch) wonton wrappers

4 cups baby spinach leaves

2 cups black beans, drained and rinsed

1 cup mozzarella cheese, shredded

1 heaping tablespoon ground cumin

Kosher salt and freshly ground black pepper to taste

Here's How

Line a baking sheet with parchment paper and two layers of paper towels. Set aside. In a large bowl, combine the spinach, beans, ground cumin, salt, pepper and cheeses. Toss to combine and disperse the spices evenly among the beans and spinach. Set aside.

On a clean work surface, lay the wonton wrappers flat in diamond shapes, with a point of the wrapper facing you at the 6 o'clock position. Working in batches of 4 to 5 at a time, spoon a heaping tablespoon of filling onto the wrapper just above the 6 o'clock point. Be sure to stuff with a balanced amount of cheese beans and spinach. Fold the bottom point of the wrapper up and over the filling and roll slightly; fold the 9 o'clock and 3 o'clock points to meet in the middle over the 6 o'clock corner.

Dip your finger in a little clean water and dab the 12 o'clock portion of the wrapper; roll the whole wrapper away from you toward 12 o'clock—sort of like a burrito—pressing gently to seal at the end. Set the rolled wonton wrapper on the prepared baking sheet, seam-side down. Continue to roll the remaining wrappers.

Heat the oil in a large saucepan on medium heat. When oil is at 350 °F, gently place a few of the egg rolls inside the hot oil and cook while carefully turning the wonton wrapper, cooking on all surface areas until browned and crispy. Remove from hot oil and set on paper towels to drain. Allow to cool, and serve with a sour cream dipping sauce or eat plain.

Makes approximately 2 dozen

~*Time-Saving Tip: Can be made up to 2 weeks in advance and stored in an airtight container in the freezer.*

Umami Meatball Patty Sliders

Something about miniature food just makes me happy. Sliders are perfect for little hands, and the kids will love feeling autonomous with their own burger.

You'll Need

1 pound ground beef (preferably chuck)

1 pound ground sausage

1/2 cup panko or other bread crumbs

1/4 cup whole milk

1 egg

1 carrot, peeled and root removed

4 cloves garlic, minced

1/2 small yellow onion, peeled, root removed

1 shallot, cleaned, root removed

Kosher salt and freshly ground black pepper

1/2 cup Parmesan cheese, finely grated

1 cup mozzarella cheese, grated large

3 tablespoons extra virgin olive oil

3 cups marinara, homemade or healthy store-bought option

2 dozen soft mini dinner rolls, sliced

Here's How

In the bowl of your food processor, combine the carrot, garlic, onion, shallot, and parsley. Blitz until fine and almost a liquid state. In a large bowl, combine the beef and pork until incorporated. Add the garlic and onion mixture from the food processor to the ground meat. Add the egg and the milk, and salt and pepper to taste. Toss with clean hands until well combined. Add the bread crumbs and roll into large, palm-size balls. Please the meatballs onto a prepared baking sheet and flatten with your hand or the bottom of a clean plastic drinking cup until they all look like mini 3-inch burgers. Set aside.

In a large high-sided sauté pan, heat 2 tablespoons olive oil over medium heat. Add the patties and brown, about 2 minutes on each side. Do this in a few batches. Once all the meatballs are browned, move them close together and gently pour in the marina sauce and the stock.

Simmer uncovered for 20 to 30 minutes. When ready to serve, split the dinner rolls and sprinkle some mozzarella on the bottom halves. Top each with a meatball patty.

Makes about 2 dozen mini sliders

~*An umami recipe*

~*Time-Saving Tip: Prepare the meatball patties ahead of time. Freeze individually on a sheet pan and, once frozen, put them all together in an airtight container. Use as needed.*

Chicken Basil Meatballs with Angel Hair Pasta

There's something about a picky eater and angel hair pasta— they just seem to couple well together.

You'll Need

Olive oil cooking spray
2 cups baby spinach
1 pound lean ground chicken
3 cloves garlic, minced
1 large egg, lightly beaten
3/4 cup whole grain bread crumbs
1/4 cup feta cheese, crumbled
1 tablespoon fresh basil leaves, finely chopped
Sea salt and freshly ground black pepper to taste
1 pound angel hair pasta, cooked
2–4 ounces butter, melted
Parmesan cheese to taste

Here's How

Preheat oven to 450 °F. Spritz a large baking dish with healthy oil cooking spray.

In a steamer basket over simmering water, steam baby spinach until wilted, about 1 to 2 minutes. Allow to cool, gently squeezing out any excess moisture; chop and set aside.

In a large bowl, combine the raw ground chicken, minced garlic cloves, lightly beaten large egg, whole grain bread crumbs, crumbled feta cheese, finely chopped fresh basil leaves, spinach, and salt and pepper to taste. Mix well to combine. Use your hands to form mixture into 12 balls.

Transfer to prepared baking dish and bake for 15 to 20 minutes, or until golden brown and no longer pink inside.

Bring a large pot of salted water to a boil over high heat. Add the pasta and cook until tender but still firm to the bite, stirring occasionally, about 3 to 4 minutes. Drain and toss with melted butter and Parmesan cheese, add basil and meatballs.

Makes approximately 6 to 8 servings

~An umami recipe

My Additive-Free Homemade Macaroni and Cheese

My children grew up on this recipe and now prepare it themselves. When they were little, I would add fresh peas and tell them the recipe was called Mac and Sneeze. Not so appetizing, but they certainly had a good laugh and gobbled it up.

You'll Need

1 pound elbow macaroni, cooked, drained and tossed in olive oil

3 tablespoons olive oil

1/2 cup sweet cream unsalted butter

1/2 cup all-purpose or gluten-free flour

1–2 cups good quality chicken or vegetable stock

1–1½ cups cream, whole milk, or nut milk

8–10 ounces cheddar cheese, shredded

1/2 teaspoon ground cayenne pepper

1/2 teaspoon ground nutmeg

1 teaspoon kosher salt

1 teaspoon crushed red pepper (optional)

1/4–1/2 cup Parmesan cheese

Chopped chives or parsley, for garnish (optional)

Here's How

In a large saucepan on low heat, melt the butter and flour together to make a thick paste; chefs call this *roux*. Continue to stir and cook the raw flour, but don't brown—about 3 to 4 minutes. This will become the thickening agent to your cheese sauce.

Combine cream with the stock. When roux is thick, combine the liquids and pour in a steady steam into the pan while whisking out the lumps. Add more liquid as you stir to smooth out to a mac-and-cheese consistency. Don't add all the liquid.

Always check for consistency. If it is too thick, add more; if it is getting too runny, cut back.

The key is to work fast over very low heat. The sauce will get tight and you'll think you've made a mistake. Keep going! Keep whisking at a steady pace. It's okay to take the pan off the heat if you think it's cooking too fast. Once you have a good consistency, add the cheese, salt and spices. Combine well. Adjust liquid if necessary. You will know it's ready when it coats the back of a spoon and you can run your finger through it and the line your finger leaves in the sauce stays clean.

If you're using additional ingredients such as red pepper flakes and Parmesan, add them now. Add the cooked elbow macaroni. Stir to combine. Serve warm!

Makes approximately 6 to 8 servings

~*Time-Saving Tip: Prepare the macaroni a day ahead. Drain and toss with a little oil to keep from sticking. Refrigerate airtight until ready to use. You can also make the sauce up to 1 week in advance and store in the refrigerator until ready to use.*

Popcorn Halibut

I love this flaky, delicate white fish, and cooking it in the pan only takes a few minutes. The popcorn is a great food pairing, and the kids just love the novelty. This recipe has been a family favorite for years.

You'll Need

2–4 (6-ounce) halibut fillets

2 tablespoons butter

1/2 cup fresh popped popcorn, for garnish

Popcorn Compound Butter (see recipe below)

Kosher salt and pepper

Few sprigs of fresh parsley, finely chopped, for garnish

Here's How

Preheat the oven 350 °F. Pop popcorn and set aside. Collect at least 1/4 cup un-popped, cooked kernels from the bottom of the popcorn popper or pan. Set aside. Heat a medium oven-safe sauté pan with 2 tablespoons butter. Melt the butter slowly, careful not to brown. When the butter is melted, turn heat up to medium-high to get the pan hot.

Pat fish dry with paper towels and season well with salt and pepper. Place fish in the hot pan and cook until the fish has a nice, rich, brown caramelized crust, about 2 to 4 minutes.

Gently turn the fish over and cook an additional 2 minutes. Careful not to burn the butter; add additional butter if needed. Tilt the pan, gather the buttery sauce in a large spoon, and bathe the fish until it is almost cooked through. Repeat bathing for 1 to 2 minutes and place the oven-safe pan in the oven to complete the fish. You can tell if the fish is cooked through by pressing on the center of the fillet and feeling for firmness or if the fish is no longer opaque—about 3 to 5 minutes, until the fish reaches 120 °F.

When fish is completely cooked through, bathe it one more

time with the warm pan sauce, plate, and immediately top with a ½-inch disc of popcorn butter and popcorn kernel dust left over from butter recipe. Sprinkle chopped parsley and 10 to 12 popcorn pieces on the fish and the surrounding plate.

Popcorn Compound Butter

Make sure you use the un-popped kernels left at the bottom of your popcorn pot after making a batch of popcorn. You will love the nutty caramel flavor the kernels add to the sweet creamy butter.

You'll Need

4 ounces unsalted butter, room temperature

1 clove garlic, cleaned

1/4 cup fresh parsley leaves

1/4 cup un-popped cooked popcorn kernels

1/4 teaspoon salt

Pinch of ground white pepper

Here's How

Place salt and un-popped cooked popcorn kernels in a food processor and process until reduced to fine dust. Remove and set aside one heaping tablespoon of popcorn kernel dust for halibut garnish.

Place softened butter in a food processer mixing bowl with the popcorn dust. Add the salt, pepper, garlic and parsley, and blitz until thoroughly combined, forming a paste. Place compound butter on a sheet of plastic wrap. Shape into a log and twist the ends to seal. Place butter in the refrigerator to harden, at least 30 minutes. When ready to use, bring closer to room temperature.

Makes approximately 4 to 5 ounces

Little Lulu's Lemon Basil Meatballs

This recipe was designed for a weeklong culinary camp at my school, Kids Culinary Adventures, located in the San Francisco Bay Area. It was inspired by my first eBook, *Learning with Little Lulu Lemon*, a fun activity guide I wrote with homeschooling expert Diane Flynn Keith of *Homefires*. The lemony basil meatballs instantly became such a big hit that they have organically become a favorite signature dish. This recipe has simple, clean flavors.

You'll Need

1 pound freshly ground lean chicken

Juice and zest of 3 lemons

1/2 teaspoon kosher salt

1/2 teaspoon freshly ground black pepper

1/8 teaspoon ground cayenne pepper

1/4 bunch fresh flat-leaf parsley leaves

5–8 large fresh basil leaves

1 small white onion, diced

2 cloves garlic, cleaned

1 egg

1/3 cup soft bread crumbs

2 tablespoons olive oil

2 tablespoons unsalted butter

Lemony Butter Garlic Sauce (see recipe below)

Here's How

Preheat the oven to 350 °F. Line a cookie sheet with foil and nonstick spray. Set aside. Set basil leaves aside.

In the bowl of your food processor, add the lemon zest, lemon juice, salt, pepper, cayenne, parsley, garlic and onion. Process to a liquid paste.

In a large bowl, combine the ground chicken and all the ingredients from food processor; add the egg and the bread crumbs. Mix thoroughly with clean hands. Cut basil and add. Combine well and shape into ½-inch to 1-inch meatballs.

In a large skillet, heat the olive oil and butter over medium-high heat. When the butter has melted, add the meatballs. Do not crowd the pan or the meatballs will steam and not brown well. Allow to brown, turning gently, until browned and cooked through, about 5 minutes total.

Transfer to the prepared baking sheet and place in the oven for an additional 10 minutes until cooked through and golden brown.

While meatballs are in the oven, make the lemon garlic sauce.

Look for meatballs to have an internal temperature of 140 °F and for juices from the meatballs to run clear; allow to rest. Serve meatballs with pasta, topped with lemony butter garlic sauce.

Makes approximately 16 meatballs

~Time-Saving Tip: Make meatballs ahead and freeze on a sheet pan. Once individually frozen, place in an airtight container and use as needed. You can also make the lemon sauce ahead and freeze in ice cube trays. Use accordingly.

Lemony Butter Garlic Sauce

This sauce is fresh, delicious and easy to make. Made to pair with my Basil Lemon Meatballs, although it also tastes great tossed with pasta and Parmesan cheese!

You'll Need

8 ounces unsalted butter

2 tablespoons good quality olive oil

Juice of 4 lemons

1 clove garlic, minced to paste

Pinch of garlic salt

4 large basil leaves, chopped last minute

2–4 sprigs flat-leaf Italian parsley leaves

Salt and pepper to taste

Here's How

In a small skillet over low heat, melt the butter. Add the garlic and cook until fragrant, about 1 minute. Add the parsley, lemon juice, and garlic. Continue to cook over medium heat until warmed through. Season with garlic salt, salt and pepper. Mince the basil and parsley together at the very last minute, add to the sauce, and swirl in the heat of the pan to release flavor.

Adjust seasoning to your preference. Spoon the topping over the meatballs or toss over pasta. Serve immediately.

Makes approximately 1 cup

~Time-Saving Tip: Make ahead and place inside ice cube trays and freeze. Once frozen, remove into an airtight container and use as needed. Melts and seasons right in the pan!

Shrimp Noodle Lettuce Cups

You'll Need

1 head butter or iceberg lettuce

1 pound large shrimp, peeled and deveined, salt and peppered

1/2 onion, diced large

1 clove garlic, peeled, left whole and smashed

Salt and pepper

1 tablespoon olive oil

1 avocado, sliced into strips

½ English cucumber, peeled and sliced into strips

2 scallions, cleaned and diagonally sliced

½ bunch cilantro

1 medium carrot, peeled and cut into matchsticks

1/4–1/2 pound vermicelli noodles

Black sesame seeds, for garnish (optional)

Quick and Easy Peanut Dipping Sauce (see recipe below)

Here's How

Cook the vermicelli according to package directions, drain, and toss in a little olive oil to keep the noodles from sticking together. When ready to serve, toss the noodles in 3/4 of the peanut sauce, reserving some for topping. Once the noodles are cooled, add to an airtight container and place in the refrigerator.

Rinse and pat the shrimp dry, season with salt and pepper, and set aside. In a large nonstick skillet over medium-low heat, heat the oil. Once oil is warmed, add the onions and garlic.

Cook the onions and garlic until they are translucent and have flavored the oil. Add the shrimp and sauté on medium-high heat, stirring until the shrimp turns pink, about 1 to 2 minutes.

Don't overcook them or they will turn rubbery. Remove from heat, set aside, cool and chill in the refrigerator.

While the noodles and shrimp are chilling, cut the cucumber and carrot into thin matchstick pieces. Set aside and keep moist with a wet paper towel. Cut avocado slices right before you serve the lettuce cups. Avocados will turn brown if they sit out too long.

Using lettuce leaves that closely resemble a bowl, sprinkle black sesame seeds and then fan out a few slices of avocado on the inside curve of the lettuce bowl. Add carrots and cucumber matchsticks. Add sliced scallions, two cooked, chilled shrimp, and a few cilantro leaves. Top with about 1/8 to 1/4 cup of noodles that have been tossed in peanut sauce.

Drizzle with a small amount of additional peanut sauce, roll up like a burrito, and place on a serving dish seam-side down. Serve with additional peanut sauce on the side for dipping. Vary these lettuce cups by adding glass noodles or cooked rice or substituting cooked chicken, beef or tofu for the shrimp.

These rolls are great for bento boxes, but note that you should never dress lettuce or veggies until you're ready to serve. The acidity of dressings will wilt these ingredients if held for a long period. Serve the sauce on the side if not served immediately.

Makes approximately 12 lettuce cups

~An umami recipe

~Time-Saving Tip: All items can be made ahead and kept in the refrigerator for up to 1 day before assembly

Quick and Easy Peanut Dipping Sauce

Kids love anything peanut-ty. If your child tolerates nuts, I'd slather this sauce on grilled chicken right before it comes off the grill, too.

You'll Need

1/4–1/2-inch nugget fresh ginger, peeled

2 cloves garlic, peeled and root ball removed

1 cup creamy peanut butter

2–3 tablespoons reduced-sodium soy sauce

2 tablespoons sesame oil

Juice of 2 large limes

1 teaspoon light brown sugar, packed

1–2 teaspoons honey

1/4 teaspoon ground cayenne pepper

Lukewarm water

Kosher salt and freshly ground black pepper to taste

Here's How

In the bowl of your food processor, add the fresh ginger and garlic. Blitz into a paste, about 30 seconds to a minute. Add soy sauce, lime juice, brown sugar, honey, and cayenne, and process again. Add peanut butter and continue to blend, adding water by tablespoon if the sauce is too thick. Process until smooth and sauce like. Adjust seasoning with salt and pepper. Transfer to an airtight container and chill.

Makes approximately 1 cup

~An umami recipe

~Time-Saving Tip: Peanut sauce can be made up to 1 week ahead of time.

Wenonalani's Cashew Chicken Lanai

You'll Need

2–6 tablespoons cooking oil

4 boneless, skinless chicken breasts, cut into strips

1 large yellow onion, julienne-sliced

5 large cloves garlic, cleaned and smashed

2 cups broccoli florets, cleaned and separated into bite-size pieces

1 cup snap peas

1/2 cup chicken stock

1/2 cup cashew nuts

1 teaspoon garlic salt

Salt and pepper to taste

1 bunch scallions, diagonally sliced

¼-inch-thick, coin-size slice fresh ginger

1 can bamboo shoots, drained

1 can baby whole corn, drained

4 slices canned pineapple rings, grilled (grilling optional)

4 cups white or brown rice, steamed

1 cup **Pineapple Carrot Stir-Fry Sauce**, divided in half (see recipe below)

Sesame seeds, for garnish

Here's How

Season the chicken strips with garlic salt and pepper; toss in 1/2 cup pineapple stir-fry sauce. Set aside.

Heat a few tablespoons of oil in a stir-fry pan, add smashed garlic, and swirl to season until the garlic is golden brown.

Remove the garlic and discard. Add the seasoned chicken, discarding any remaining marinade sauce. Stir-fry the chicken until it turns white and cooks halfway, not completely brown, about 2 to 3 minutes. Remove the chicken to a plate and set aside, reserving its juices.

Add another 1 to 2 tablespoons of oil to the stir-fry pan and add the ginger and the broccoli. Stir-fry for about 2 minutes until the broccoli is a vibrant green and just beginning to cook through. Add the onions. Stir-fry until the onions are fragrant but still crunchy, about a minute.

Return the chicken to the pan and cook until browned. Add chicken stock, snap peas, bamboo shoots and baby corn. Stir-fry until liquid is almost evaporated. Add the cashew nuts and do a few quick stirs, about 1 to 2 minutes. Do not overcook.

Add the remaining 1/2 cup of pineapple stir-fry sauce, and stir continuously until the chicken is cooked and well coated with the sauce, about 1 additional minute. Add salt and pepper to taste. Top with sesame seeds. Serve with steamed rice and grilled pineapple.

Makes approximately 4 to 6 servings.

~An umami recipe

Pineapple Carrot Stir-Fry Sauce

You'll Need

1 (15-ounce) can pineapple cubes, ¼ cup juice reserved

1 small onion, diced large

1 large carrot, peeled and cleaned, roughly chopped

2 cloves garlic, cleaned and smashed

Zest and juice of 1 lime

1/8–1/4-inch-thick knob fresh ginger, sliced into coins, skin removed

1/4 teaspoon ground ginger

1/8 teaspoon ground cinnamon

1/4 teaspoon crushed red pepper (optional)

1/2 cup low-sodium ponzu or soy sauce

1/4 cup honey

2 teaspoons cornstarch

Kosher salt and freshly ground black pepper

Here's How

Place all ingredients except the water and the cornstarch in the bowl of your food processor. Process all the ingredients to a liquid. Add the liquid to a medium saucepan and cook on low heat for 8 to 10 minutes. Season with salt and pepper.

Mix 1/4 cup water with the cornstarch. Place the cornstarch mixture into the saucepan. Stir until sauce thickens and coats the back of a spoon. Remove from heat and cool. Store sauce in a jar or squeeze bottle. Seal airtight. Use on stir-fry chicken or beef with vegetables for a quick weeknight meal.

Makes approximately 1 quart of sauce

~An umami recipe

~Time-Saving Tip: Make sauce ahead and freeze in ice cube trays. Once frozen, pop into a freezer-safe bag and use individually for quick midweek meals

Dakota's Spicy Chili with Toasted Cumin Crème and Avocado Salsa

You'll Need

1/4 cup plus 2 tablespoons olive oil, divided

2 pounds tender cuts beef, cut into 1/2-inch cubes

4 tablespoons flour

1–2 teaspoons kosher salt

Freshly ground black pepper

1 large onion, medium diced

4 cloves garlic, finely chopped

3 tablespoons ancho chili powder

1 tablespoon chili powder

1 tablespoon ground cumin

1 teaspoon ground white pepper

4 cups beef stock, homemade or good quality premade

1 (12-ounce) can tomato puree

1 tablespoon chipotle pepper puree, canned or fresh

2 tablespoons honey

2 (12-ounce) cans black beans, rinsed, drained, and cooked

1 (12-ounce) can kidney beans, rinsed, drained, and cooked

Juice of 2 large limes

Toasted Cumin Crème (see recipe below)

Avocado Cucumber Salsa (see page 240)

Here's How

In a large Dutch oven or heavy-bottomed stockpot, heat oil over medium-low heat. Season the beef with salt and black pepper and toss with flour. Increase heat to medium; add the meat and brown on all sides. Once brown, remove and transfer the meat to a plate. Add 2 tablespoons olive oil. Heat. Add the onions to the pan and cook until soft and somewhat translucent. Add the garlic and cook for 2 minutes, careful not to burn the garlic—it will cook fast.

Return the beef to the pot and add the beef stock, the ancho powder, chili powder and cumin, and cook an additional 2 minutes. Add the tomatoes, tomato puree, chipotle puree and honey and bring to a boil. Reduce the heat to medium, do not cover the pot, and simmer for 60 to 90 minutes or until beef is tender. Add the beans and continue cooking for 15 minutes. Remove from the heat, add the lime juice, and adjust the seasonings with salt and black pepper to taste. Serve with a dollop of toasted cumin crème and avocado salsa. Chili goes well with **Little Lulu Lemon's Cornbread** (see page 241).

Makes approximately 8 to 10 servings

~An umami recipe

Dakota's Toasted Cumin Crème

You'll Need

1 tablespoon cumin seeds

1 teaspoon ground cumin

1/2 teaspoon garlic salt

1 pint plain Greek yogurt

Kosher salt and ground white pepper to taste

Here's How

Place the cumin seeds in a small sauté pan over medium heat. Toast until lightly golden brown. Be careful not to burn them; this process goes fast. In a small bowl, mix the Greek yogurt, toasted cumin seeds, ground cumin and the garlic salt, and season with salt and white pepper to taste.

Makes approximately 2 cups.

Dakota's Avocado Cucumber Salsa

You'll Need

2 large firm but ripe avocados, pitted and medium diced

1/2 small shallot, finely diced

1 serrano chili, finely diced (optional)

Juice from 1/4 of a lemon

1/2 teaspoon soy sauce

1 tablespoon fresh cilantro leaves, finely chopped

1 large English cucumber, cold, peeled, deseeded, and diced small

Kosher salt and ground white pepper to taste

1/2 teaspoon celery salt

Here's How

In a small bowl, combine the diced avocado, shallot, chili, cilantro and lime juice, and season with salt and white pepper to taste. Toss gently so as not to smash the avocado dice. Add cucumber and celery salt and toss again. Serve immediately. Serve with Dakota's spicy chili with toasted cumin crème and avocado salsa; recipes above.

Makes approximately 1½ cups.

~An umami recipe

Little Lulu Lemon's Cornbread

You'll Need

1 stick butter, melted

2/3 cup white sugar

2 eggs, beaten

1½ cups cornmeal

1 cup canned sweet white or yellow corn, drained

1/2 cup all-purpose flour

1 teaspoon salt

2 teaspoons baking powder

1½ cups buttermilk

Here's How

Preheat the oven to 450 °F. Grease an 8-inch square pan. Combine all ingredients in a large bowl and mix well until very few lumps remain. Pour the batter into the prepared pan. Bake for 30 to 40 minutes or until a toothpick inserted in the center comes out clean. This cornbread is moist and delicious!

Makes approximately 10 to 12 servings

Chicken Drumsticks Dijonnaise

You'll Need

1–2 teaspoons ground cumin

2 tablespoons extra virgin olive oil

3 pounds chicken drumsticks (about 8)

Kosher salt and freshly ground black pepper

1 onion, finely sliced

4 cloves garlic, minced

1½ cups chicken stock

2 tablespoons whole grain mustard

3 tablespoons crème fraiche or sour cream

2 teaspoons fresh tarragon, chopped

Here's How

Heat the olive oil until shimmering. Season the chicken drumsticks with salt and pepper. Place the chicken in skillet and cook, turning often, until nicely brown, about 10 minutes. Add onions and garlic. Cook about 3 minutes, stirring.

Add chicken stock and cumin. Bring to a boil. Cover, reduce heat to low, and cook until done, about 30 minutes. Remove chicken and set aside. In a bowl, whisk together the mustard, crème fraiche and tarragon. Add to pan and stir until thickened. Return the chicken to pan and blanket with the sauce! *Ooooh la la*!

Chicago Joe's Potato Soup with Almond Milk

All children seem to love mashed potatoes. Here is a spinoff to that love affair in a healthier, non-dairy soup version.

You'll Need

2 tablespoons olive oil

2 large leeks

1 medium onion, chopped

2 cloves fresh garlic

1 medium carrot, thinly sliced

4 large baking potatoes, peeled and cut into 1-inch chunks

1/2 pound nitrate-free bacon, cut into 1-inch pieces

1–2 teaspoons ground white pepper to taste (depending on how spicy you want your soup)

1–2 teaspoons salt to taste

4 cups chicken stock

1–2 cups almond milk (depending on how thick you like your soup)

Soy sauce and additional ground white pepper to taste

Chives or scallions, chopped, for garnish

Cheddar cheese, grated, for garnish

Here's How

Remove roots, outer leaves, and tops from leeks, leaving only white part. Cut white part in half lengthwise. Rinse with cold water between the leeks' layers, looking for any additional dirt or sand. Drain and cut leek halves into ½-inch to 1-inch pieces, and set aside.

Peel and cut potatoes. Set aside in a large bowl of water—soaking peeled potatoes in water will prevent them from browning while you prepare the remaining ingredients. This is a white soup, so we try not to brown anything.

Clean and chop the onion, garlic, and carrot; set aside. Meanwhile, in an 8-quart saucepan, cook bacon until crisp. Drain on paper towels. Crumble bacon; set aside. Cook leeks, onion, garlic and carrot in bacon drippings over medium heat for 3 minutes, adding 2 tablespoons of the olive oil to prevent sticking; cook a few more minutes until the onion begins to look translucent, stirring occasionally, careful not to overly brown any of the ingredients. Add potatoes to the pot, discarding the soaking liquid.

Add broth to cover all ingredients, scraping the pan to loosen any slightly brown particles on the bottom. Add salt. Cook until the carrot and potatoes are cooked through, about 30 minutes; cooking time will depend on the size of the carrot and potato chunks. When potatoes and carrot are cooked through, submerge an immersion hand blender and blend all ingredients into liquid, or use a standing blender and work in batches. Add white pepper and taste. Adjust seasoning to your liking with soy and additional white pepper if needed. After the mixture is pureed, return to the pot.

Gradually add almond milk, stirring until smoothed to a soup-like consistency. Blend again after any white pepper additions. Cook uncovered an additional 10 minutes; do not boil. Stir occasionally until thoroughly heated. If you prefer your soup at a thinner consistency, add chicken stock or water during the blending process. Remember to adjust the seasoning after any additions of liquid.

Serve warm with crumbled bacon, grated cheddar cheese, and chives for toppings.

Makes 8 to 10 servings

~Time-Saving Tip: Recipe calls for a handheld immersion blender. You can also cool soup and blend in a standing blender or food processor.

~An umami recipe

Gab's Southwest Corn Chowder

You'll Need

1 pound bacon, cut in 1/4-inch strips

1 yellow onion, diced small

2 large carrots, diced small

2 celery ribs, diced small

1/2 red bell pepper, diced into ¼-inch pieces

1/2 pound Yukon Gold or other yellow-fleshed potato, peeled, diced small

2 quarts good quality chicken broth

2 sprigs fresh thyme

3 cups corn (from about 6 ears; or frozen, thawed and drained)

1 cup heavy cream or substitute, warmed

1 tablespoon kosher salt

1–2 teaspoons ground white pepper

1 cup cheddar cheese, grated

Crushed red pepper to taste (optional)

Kosher salt and pepper to taste

Here's How

In a 6 or 8-quart heavy-bottomed Dutch oven or stockpot, cook the bacon pieces over moderate heat, stirring frequently until crisp, about 5 to 8 minutes. Transfer the cooked bacon with a slotted spoon to paper towels to drain. Set aside. Reduce heat and add the onions, carrots, and celery to the bacon drippings, and cook, stirring, until the onions are softened, about 5 additional minutes.

Add potatoes, broth, and thyme sprigs. Cover and bring to a simmer until potatoes are tender, about 15 minutes. Add 2/3 of the corn and the cream, stirring uncovered for about 10 minutes. Add salt and pepper to adjust seasoning. Remove thyme sprigs and place half of the corn chowder into a blender or food processor with cooking liquid, or use an immersion blender and blend until smooth. Add additional stock if needed to create a soup-like consistency.

Return the mixture to the cooking pot. Repeat the blending process with the remaining chowder mixture. Add remaining fresh corn and stir in red bell peppers. Heat through and serve warm. Garnish with bacon and cheddar cheese.

Makes approximately 8 to 10 servings

Dinosaur-as Teriyaki Drumettes

You'll Need

12 chicken drumsticks, room temperature

2 green onions, diagonally sliced

2 cloves garlic, minced

1/2 cup low-sodium soy sauce

2/3 cup water

1 tablespoon rice vinegar

2 tablespoons honey

4 tablespoons brown sugar

1 teaspoon ground ginger

2 tablespoons cornstarch

1/4–1/2 cup cold water

Kosher salt and freshly ground black pepper to taste

Sesame seeds

Here's How

Preheat the oven to 375 °F. Prepare a baking sheet with parchment paper lightly spritzed with nonstick cooking spray, or a silicone baking mat, and set aside. Run the chicken drumsticks under running water and pat dry. Grasp the skin at the wide end of each drumstick and pull it down to remove it. Discard the skin. Place the skinless drumsticks in a large mixing bowl, add salt and pepper, and toss.

In a small bowl or a coffee cup, combine the cornstarch and the 1/2 cup cold water, using a fork mix the lumps out. Set aside.

In a small saucepan, combine the remaining ingredients except for the cornstarch and water slurry. Stir constantly on medium-low heat until sugar crystals are melted, then add the cornstarch and water mixture. Continue to stir on medium-low heat and bring to a slow boil.

Once the sauce comes to a boil, it will begin to thicken. Reduce heat immediately and continue to heat until it reaches a maple syrup consistency. Add water if it becomes too thick. Ideally, the glaze will be ready when it coats the back of a spoon and you can run your finger though it without the sauce swelling back into the line you made with your fingertip. Cool until just warm. Drizzle sauce onto the drumsticks in a bowl, reserving 1/3 of the sauce. Toss to coat well.

Place the drumsticks on the prepared baking sheet, making sure they are evenly separated. Bake for 40 to 50 minutes. Test the drumsticks for doneness by cutting into the thickest part with a knife to see if the chicken has lost its pink color and the juices run clear, or if it has reached an internal temperature of 165 °F.

Brush the remaining glaze onto the chicken the last 5 minutes of baking time. Sprinkle with sesame seeds and serve with stir-fry veggies and **Keoni's Mango Sticky Rice** (see recipe on the right).

Makes 10 to 12 drumsticks

~*An umami recipe*

Keoni's Coconut Mango Sticky Rice

This recipe is lots of work and could take up to a day to prepare. It also requires a few kitchen tools that you might not use on a daily basis. But once you try this recipe, you will be hooked. The kids love it, and sticky rice is also a great addition to dessert or accompaniment to grilled foods.

You'll Need

1½ cups Thai sticky rice (*khao niao*)

Water to cover and soak rice overnight

1 (19-ounce) can unsweetened coconut milk

1/4–1/2 cup sugar or sugar substitute

1/4 teaspoon salt

2 teaspoons cornstarch

2 mangos, peeled, sliced, and diced

Here's How

In a large bowl, combine the rice and enough water to cover by 2 inches. Cover and soak the rice for at least 6 and up to 24 hours. Line a colander with a double layer of damp cheesecloth. Spritz the inside of the cheesecloth with nonstick spray. Set aside.

In a stovetop steamer, bring enough water to a boil to steam for 30 minutes. Spritz the inside of the steamer with nonstick cooking spray. Drain the rice of its soaking liquid. Do not rinse. Once almost all the liquid is drained off the cheesecloth, tie up the ends to close. Squeeze any excessive liquid from the cheesecloth when you pick up the ends.

Place the drained cheesecloth bag containing the rice into the prepared steamer rack. Flatten into a disk as much as you can without compromising the closure of the bag. Check the positioning of the cheesecloth bag in the steamer and make sure the rice is not touching any of the steaming liquid.

Reduce the steaming heat to medium-low, cover, and steam until rice is tender, about 20 to 30 minutes. While rice is steaming, prepare the coconut milk sauce.

Shake the container of coconut milk before opening. Add coconut milk to a medium saucepan over medium-low heat, reserving 1/4 cup.

Add the sugar and salt and bring to a simmer, stirring until the sugar dissolves, about 1 minute. Add more sugar if you would like sweeter rice. Taste the mixture and adjust flavoring to your liking.

In the meantime, combine the cornstarch and the remaining coconut milk. Add the cornstarch mixture to the saucepan and bring the coconut milk close to a quick boil, making sure the milk and sugar mix does not burn or boil over. Once you reach a boil, reduce heat, and stir constantly the last few moments as the sauce begins to thicken. You will know it is done when it coats the back of a spoon. Remove from heat and cool slightly.

While sauce is cooling, carefully remove rice from cheesecloth bag into a medium high-sided mixing bowl. With a plastic or wooden paddle or spoon, spread the rice in the bowl to release heat and break it apart. The rice will be very sticky on the cheesecloth. Remove it the best you can. *The steam from rice will be hot and can burn! Be careful!*

Pour thickened coconut milk mixture over the rice, mix well, cover and set aside until liquid is absorbed, about 30 minutes. Top with diced mangos.

Serve the rice with the grilled **Little Lil's Grilled Ponzu Chicken Skewers** (see recipe below) or **Dinosaur-us Teriyaki Drumettes** (see page 247). The rice dish can be kept covered at room temperature for 6 to 8 hours. Do not refrigerate or the rice will harden.

Makes approximately 4 to 6 servings

Little Lil's Grilled Ponzu Chicken Skewers

Ponzu is a type of Japanese dipping sauce made from orange juice, sake, sugar, soy sauce and red pepper, and is found in most markets today, or you can purchase it online.

You'll Need

2 large shallots, peeled and roughly chopped

2-inch piece fresh ginger, peeled and smashed

4 cloves garlic, cleaned and smashed

1/4 cup soy sauce

2/3 cup ponzu sauce

3 tablespoons brown sugar

2 tablespoons honey

1/4 cup green onions, roughly chopped

1/4 cup peanut or liquid coconut oil or canola

3–4 tablespoons warm water

Salt and pepper

Black sesame seeds (optional)

12 boneless, skinless chicken breast or thighs, cut in bite-size pieces

6–8 long skewers, soaked in water for 30 minutes

Here's How

Place the shallots, garlic, soy sauce, ponzu, sugar and honey in the bowl of your food processor or blender and blend until smooth. Add the green onion and oil and blend until combined. Add a few tablespoons of warm water if the sauce is too thick. Season with black pepper to taste, and blend again. Add the smashed ginger coin to the marinade. Allow marinade to sit for about 20 minutes up to overnight. Reserve a 1/2 cup of marinade in a separate small bowl. Set aside.

Season the chicken with salt and pepper and place in a gallon-size food storage bag. Pour the marinade over the chicken and let marinate at room temperature for 60 minutes. Preheat a grill to high. Remove the chicken from the marinade, dry skewers, and thread the chicken on the skewers. Discard any leftover marinade that the chicken was soaking in, including the smashed ginger.

Check temperature of the grill and oil the grates immediately before use. I use an organic spray, and I always stand a few steps away from the grill because the spray will ignite a flame. Be careful.

Using tongs, place chicken skewers on grill for 3 to 4 minutes on each side, or until cooked through, showing no pink, and the juices run clear and internal temperatures reach 165 °F. The last 2 minutes of cooking, lightly brush remaining sauce on chicken. Remove from the grill and sprinkle with black sesame seeds. Serve with **Keoni's Coconut Mango Sticky Rice** (see page 249) and eat with your fingers.

Makes 6 to 8 servings

~An umami recipe

~Time-Saving Tip: Marinade can be made up to 1 week in advance and stored airtight.

Popcorn Fish Fingers

You'll Need

4–6 pieces wild-caught Dover sole, cut lengthwise into thick strips

Kosher salt and freshly ground pepper to taste

6 cups freshly popped, buttered, and salted popcorn

2 eggs

1/4 teaspoon ground cayenne pepper

1 cup cake flour or flour of your choice, sifted

Extra virgin coconut oil

Here's How

In the bowl of your food processor, add the popcorn and blitz on high speed until the mixture is the size of small green peas. If you're using plain, unsalted popcorn, drop a generous pinch or two of salt inside the bowl.

Add the sifted flour to a shallow dish and season with salt and pepper. Set aside.

In a second shallow dish, beat the eggs with a pinch of salt, pepper and the cayenne pepper. Set aside.

Remove the popcorn from the processor and place in a third shallow dish. Line up the dishes from left to right starting with the flour mixture, following with the egg mixture, and finishing with the popcorn mixture. To the right of the popcorn mixture, place a baking sheet lined with parchment or a silicone baking mat. Preheat the oven to 375 °F. Preseason each fish fillet with salt and pepper.

Working from left to right, begin by pressing seasoned fish fillets into the seasoned flour, coating both sides. Gently shake off the excess flour, move the fish into the next container, and dip the fish fillets into the egg mixture, gently coating both sides. Last, dredge the fillet in the popcorn breading, pressing gently to thoroughly coat each side with popcorn crust.

Set coated fillets onto the prepared baking sheet. Bake immediately in a hot oven for 12 to 20 minutes, or until fish is cooked through and crust is lightly browned. Serve with fresh-made tartar sauce, warm melted butter, or homemade ranch dip.

Makes approximately 4 to 6 servings

Skinny Orange Chicken

Orange chicken is always a first choice for my kids. And parents love it, too, because it is baked and not fried.

You'll Need

- 2 cups all-purpose or gluten-free flour
- 2 large eggs, beaten
- 2 cups panko or gluten-free option
- 6 boneless, skinless chicken breasts, cut into 1-inch chunks
- Kosher salt and freshly ground black pepper
- Juice and zest of 2 oranges
- 1/3 cup low-sodium soy sauce
- 1/4 cup honey
- 2 dried chili peppers
- 2 cloves garlic, minced
- 2 teaspoons ginger, skin removed, and grated
- 2 heaping tablespoons cornstarch
- 2 cups jasmine rice, cooked
- Black or white sesame seeds, for garnish
- Sliced scallions, for garnish

Here's How

Preheat the oven to 400 °F. Line a high-sided baking sheet with parchment paper or a nonstick silicone baking sheet. Set up a dredging station with three medium shallow containers—one dish filled with the flour and seasoned with salt and pepper; another with eggs, beaten and seasoned with salt and pepper; a final container with the dry panko. Next to the last bowl, place the prepared baking sheet.

Season the chicken pieces with salt and pepper. Dredge the chicken by first pressing it in the flour. Lift to shake off any excess. Coat in the beaten eggs and finally the panko, covering thoroughly. Arrange the coated chicken on the baking sheet and bake until no longer pink, about 15 to 20 minutes.

To make the sauce, in a small saucepan over medium heat, combine the orange juice, soy sauce, honey, garlic, ginger and cornstarch. Whisk until combined. Add chili peppers and cook until thickened, about 5 minutes.

Once the chicken is baked and crispy, transfer to a large bowl and drizzle with the orange sauce. Toss well to coat. Serve with steamed rice and garnish with orange zest, sesame seeds and chopped scallions.

Makes approximately 4 to 6 servings

Vegetable Udon Noodle Soup

Kids love noodles. Udon noodles are long, thick, and satisfying—and so much fun they will rarely say no!

You'll Need

1/2 large onion, julienne-sliced

1 stalk celery, diagonally sliced

2 carrots, peeled and sliced into thin coins

1 clove garlic, smashed

Kosher salt and freshly ground pepper to taste

2 packs fresh udon noodles

1 quart beef, chicken, or vegetable stock

2 cups dashi broth (optional)

Soy sauce to taste

1 bunch green onions, sliced thin

Cilantro, parsley and basil leaves, roughly chopped, for garnish

Here's How

Add the stock, onion, celery, carrots, soy sauce, and pepper to a large stockpot on medium-low heat. Stir often and cook until the vegetables begin to soften, approximately 5 to 10 minutes. Add the fresh noodles and the dashi broth, reduce the heat to medium and allow to simmer for 5 to 8 minutes until noodles are cooked through. Once the noodles are soft but not mushy, add the cilantro, basil, parsley and green onions. Stir thoroughly.

Makes approximately 4 servings.

~An umami recipe

Fish Tacos with Tangy Savoy Cabbage Coleslaw

You'll Need

Slaw

> 1 small head savoy cabbage, shredded
>
> 1/2 red onion, very thinly sliced
>
> 1 carrot, peeled and grated
>
> 1/2 cup fresh cilantro, chopped
>
> 3 tablespoons apple cider vinegar
>
> 1 cup plain Greek yogurt
>
> 1 teaspoon honey or agave
>
> 1/2 teaspoon garlic salt
>
> Freshly ground black pepper
>
> 1/2 bunch cilantro, finely chopped
>
> 2 teaspoons poppy seeds (optional, as some picky eaters won't eat anything with black specks)
>
> Chili lime sauce (optional)

Chili Lime Sauce

> 1 cup homemade mayonnaise
>
> Juice and zest of 2 limes
>
> 1 serrano chili, stem removed (optional)
>
> 1 large clove garlic
>
> Pinch of ground cayenne pepper

Batter

> 1 cup all-purpose flour, sifted
>
> 1/2 teaspoon kosher salt
>
> 1 teaspoon freshly ground black pepper
>
> 1 teaspoon baking powder
>
> 1–2 cups soda water

Fish

6–7 pieces skinless firm white fish such as Cod, cut into 1-inch long strips

Vegetable oil for deep pan frying

Kosher salt and ground white pepper

12 (6-inch) soft corn tortillas

2 limes cut into wedges

Here's How

For the slaw: In a large bowl, toss the cabbage, red onion, cilantro, vinegar, honey, yogurt, garlic salt, pepper, cilantro and poppy seeds together. Cover with plastic-wrap and set aside in the refrigerator to chill. You can make this up to 1 day in advance.

For the chili lime sauce: In the bowl of your mini food processor, add the garlic and blitz until it becomes paste; add the serrano chilies and blitz again until paste. Add the mayonnaise and lime juice, and blend until smooth. Adjust seasoning by adding cayenne, salt, and white pepper to taste. Remove and place in an airtight container and set aside in the refrigerator. Can make up to 2 days in advance.

For the batter: In a medium bowl, combine the flour, salt, baking powder and pepper. Gradually add the soda water, whisking until the batter is smooth with no lumps. Set aside.

To assemble: In a lightly oiled pan, warm the tortillas individually on both sides until the edges are slightly brown. Lightly wrap in foil and place in a 200 °F oven with a small bowl of warm water until the fish is ready; the water will prevent the corn tortillas from becoming too dry.

In a deep skillet over medium heat, add enough vegetable oil to reach a depth of 2 inches. Heat the oil until a deep-fry thermometer registers 350 °F, or test with a small drizzle of the batter. The oil is ready when the batter sizzles in the oil.

Working in batches so as not to crowd the pan, salt and pepper the fish. Dip the fish strips in the batter and coat on both sides. Let the excess batter drip off, and then fry the fish in the hot oil until golden brown and cooked through, about 2 minutes per side. Transfer to a plate lined with paper towels to drain.

To assemble a taco, spread a tablespoon or more of the chili lime sauce onto the center of each tortilla, lay one or two pieces of the fried fish on top of the sauce, top with cold slaw, and fold over to make a soft taco. Serve with lime wedges and squeeze the fresh lime juice directly on top of the taco filling.

Makes approximately 10 to 12 tacos

Chicken Fingers with Honey Mustard Dipping Sauce

My chicken nuggets are better than theirs! (You know who I'm talking about!) Yep, I said it. Just say no to fast food and make these in 30 minutes or less!

You'll Need

6 chicken breast, sliced lengthwise in ½-inch thick pieces

2 cups plain Greek yogurt, mayonnaise or homemade ranch dressing

1 teaspoon garlic powder

1 teaspoon paprika

1 teaspoon freshly ground black pepper

1 teaspoon kosher salt

1 teaspoon Italian seasoning (if only using yogurt to coat)

1 cup crushed organic cornflake-type cereal or panko (I like it better with the cereal.)

Honey mustard sauce (see recipe below or serve with my **Homemade Ketchup**, recipe on page 103)

Here's How

In a gallon-size plastic zipper bag, add the yogurt or ranch dressing—or a combo of both. (I like ranch best!) Add the Italian seasoning if you're only using yogurt or mayonnaise.

In an additional gallon-size plastic zipper bag, add the cereal. Smash into large crumbs.

Season the chicken with the spices on the front and back. Dip into the wet ingredients to completely coat, and then dip into the dry ingredients to completely coat.

Bake at 350 °F for about 10 to 20 minutes or until cooked, turning at the midway point.

While the chicken bakes, make the honey mustard dip.

Makes approximately 6 servings

Honey Mustard Dipping Sauce

Traditionally, honey mustard dipping sauce is made with a mayonnaise base, but I've also included an alternative base.

You'll Need

1 cup mayonnaise or plain Greek yogurt

1/2 cup your child's favorite prepared mustard

1/4 cup honey

1 tablespoon apple cider vinegar

Pinch of kosher salt

Dash of cayenne pepper (optional)

Dash of Worcestershire sauce

Here's How

In a small bowl whisk all the ingredients together and store in an airtight container in the refrigerator until use.

Makes 1½ cups

~An umami recipe

~Time-Saving Tip: You can prepare the sauce up to 1 week in advance. Keep sealed airtight and refrigerated.

Mashed Potato Bombs

These mashed potato bombs are a fun way to use up any leftover mashed potatoes—or a good excuse to make more! Kids love them, and they love to dip them in homemade ketchup and ranch dressing.

You'll Need

3 cups mashed potatoes, chilled

1 cup cheddar cheese, grated

1/2 cup bacon, diced small

1 bunch chives, chopped

Freshly ground black pepper to taste

Breading

1 cup flour or gluten-free flour

2 eggs, beaten

1½ cups panko or gluten-free bread crumbs

3/4 cup Parmesan cheese, finely grated

Extra virgin coconut oil, ghee, or organic canola oil, for frying

Here's How

In a medium sauté pan, cook the bacon until crisp. Drain on a paper towel and crumble when cooled. Set aside.

In a mixing bowl, combine the mashed potatoes with the eggs, cheese, chives, and cooked and crumbled bacon. Mix to combine; cover and set aside in the refrigerator.

Prepare three breading stations: one shallow container filled with flour, one with beaten eggs and one with panko and the Parmesan cheese.

Dust your hands with flour and use a 1/2-ounce portion-control scoop to measure the balls (or a tablespoon). Pat gently to form them into balls, and roll them in your palms to get perfectly round. Immediately dust with flour again and set aside. Repeat until you have 24 flour-dusted balls.

Drop a ball into the egg mixture and use a spoon to turn it over until fully coated. Lift the potato ball out of the egg mixture with a fork. Drain any excess. Immediately drop the potato ball into the panko and cheese mixture and use another spoon to dredge it fully. Pat in any excess bread crumbs that might be falling off the ball. Set aside on your prepared baking sheet and repeat with remaining balls.

Fry in batches in hot oil over medium-high heat until golden brown on all sides, about 3 minutes. Drain on paper towels. Or bake at 400 °F for 5 to 10 minutes, or until golden brown.

Potato Leek and Pancetta Gratin

A gratin is a culinary technique for a casserole over which a rich, browned crust forms with bread crumbs or cheese. The gratin originated in French cuisine and is usually prepared in a shallow cooking vessel. The flavors are rich and delicious and very easy to prepare.

You'll Need

2 tablespoons unsalted butter

2 fresh leeks, trimmed, sliced lengthwise down the center and washed well

1½ pounds Yukon Gold potatoes, peeled

1/4–1/2 pound pancetta or center cut bacon, diced medium (optional)

1 cup heavy cream or nut milk

1/3 cup chicken or vegetable stock

2 cloves garlic, cleaned and smashed, root ball intact

2 sprigs thyme

1 bay leaf

1/4 teaspoon freshly ground nutmeg

1/4 teaspoon ground white pepper

Kosher salt and freshly ground black pepper

1 cup Gruyère cheese, grated

Here's How

Prepare a 2-quart gratin or casserole dish by generously rubbing with butter. Place on a lined, high-sided cookie sheet and set aside. Preheat oven to 350 °F.

Slice the potatoes into 1/8-inch disks. Toss with salt and pepper. Layer the rounds, slightly overlapping, from left to right or in a circle, bottom to top, in the buttered gratin dish. In a small saucepan, cook the pancetta until crispy, about 3 to 5 minutes. Drain on a paper towel. Set aside.

Cut the cleaned leeks into 1/4-inch strips. In a large skillet over medium heat, melt the butter. Add the leeks, a large pinch of salt, and a few grinds of fresh pepper. Add the thyme. Cook, stirring occasionally, until leeks are tender and golden, 5 to 7 minutes. Discard thyme sprigs and scatter the cooked leeks over the sliced potatoes.

While the leeks are cooking, heat the cream and the stock with the garlic and bay leaf in an additional saucepan. Simmer for about 5 minutes until flavors are infused in the cream. Add nutmeg and white pepper.

Sprinkle half of the pancetta on top of the cooked leeks. Pour the cream over the top. Top with the Gruyère. Cover with aluminum foil and bake for 40 to 50 minutes. Uncover and bake an additional 15 to 20 minutes until the cheese is bubbling and golden brown. Remove from oven, sprinkle with the reserved crispy pancetta, and garnish with chopped parsley.

Makes approximately 4 to 6 servings

Gold Yukons, Smashed and Baked

These potatoes go through it all. The result? Delicious!

You'll Need

12 Yukon Gold Potatoes

Olive oil

Kosher salt and freshly ground black pepper

A bouquet of assorted herbs: rosemary, thyme, herbes de Provence, parsley

Here's How

Wash the potatoes and add them to a pot of boiling water. Cook until tender, about 12 to 15 minutes depending on their size. You want the potato cooked enough to smash them but not overcooked so it won't hold its shape.

Preheat oven to 400 °F. Drizzle a foil-lined baking sheet with olive oil. Place the potatoes on the cookie sheet, leaving some room in between. With a round drinking glass, gently push each potato to smash it, careful to keep the potato in one whole piece.

After each potato is smashed, season the potatoes with garlic salt and pepper and top with chopped herbs. Drizzle the potatoes with additional olive oil. Be generous; this helps them crisp up.

Bake until brown and crispy, about 20 to 30 minutes depending on the degree of moisture in the potatoes. You might need to apply additional oven time to reach optimum crunch.

Makes approximately 4 to 6 servings

~Time-Saving Tip: Potatoes can be boiled up to 1 day ahead before baking. Bring to room temperature before smashing.

Umami Fried Garlic Rice

Rice is often cooked with other ingredients, such as vegetables, to create a dish similar to pilaf. Here is a simple version utilizing vegetables available year-round. Feel free to substitute other seasonal vegetables as desired. Soy sauce is used in this recipe to enhance umami.

You'll Need

3 tablespoons butter

1 large yellow onion, very finely chopped

2 cloves garlic, minced

2 carrots, cut same size as the onion

6 cups short-grain brown or white rice, cooked

2 eggs, beaten

½ teaspoon garlic salt

1/4 cup soy sauce

1 cup frozen green peas, cooked and held warm

Here's How

In a large wok or pan, heat the butter, add the onion, garlic and carrots, and sauté until the carrots and onions take on a brown color. Add the cooked rice and stir until the carrots and onion are incorporated into the rice. Add the beaten eggs and toss quickly to cook the egg through. Add the garlic salt and stir well, cooking the rice mixture; add the soy sauce and toss. Add the cooked peas, toss to fluff the rice up, and serve immediately.

Makes approximately 6 to 8 servings

~Time-Saving Tip: To enhance the umami flavors of this or any dish, use dashi broth instead of water.

Sweet Cauliflower and Parsnip Puree

What looks like mashed potatoes and feels like mashed potatoes but is not mashed potatoes? Cauliflower and parsnip puree! Sweet and delicious.

You'll Need

1/2 head cauliflower, stem removed and cut into 1/2-inch pieces

4 large parsnips, peeled, hard core removed, if any, and chopped into 1/2-inch thick coins

2–4 cups chicken broth

4 ounces unsalted butter, room temperature, cut into chunks

Kosher salt and ground white pepper to taste

Here's How

In a large 6 to 8-quart stockpot, bring the chicken broth to a boil. Add the cauliflower and the parsnips; bring back to a boil. Cover and reduce the heat to low for 20 minutes or until cauliflower and parsnips are tender.

Use a slotted spoon to transfer the cauliflower and parsnips to a food processor. Add 1/4 to 1/2 cup cooking liquid from the pot, along with the butter, and process until smooth and looking like mashed potatoes. Adjust your consistency with additional broth if necessary. Taste and adjust seasoning with salt and white pepper. Serve warm.

Makes approximately 4 servings

~Time-Saving Tip: You can boil the vegetables up to 2 days in advance. Store in airtight container until ready to use. Bring everything to room temperature before proceeding. Heat after puree process.

Creamy Butternut Squash Polenta

Three words: Creamy, sweet and delicious!

You'll Need

1 large butternut squash, split lengthwise, deseeded

1 cup yellow onion, very finely chopped

5 tablespoons unsalted butter, divided

3 cups chicken stock, warmed

1½–2 cups organic half and half, whole milk, or nut milk (*not* 1% or skim)

1½ teaspoons kosher salt

1/4 teaspoon ground white pepper

1 cup fine yellow cornmeal

1/2 cup Parmigiano-Reggiano or Pecorino Romano, finely grated

Here's How

Preheat the oven to 350 °F. Line a baking sheet with foil. Brush the butternut squash flesh with olive oil and a sprinkling of salt. Place flesh-side down on the foil and bake for 30 minutes or until flesh is soft.

Melt 3 tablespoons of the butter in a medium saucepan over medium-low heat. Add the onion and sauté until translucent, about 5 minutes. Do not brown.

Add the squash puree, stock, milk, salt and white pepper and bring to a boil. Reduce the heat to medium and slowly add the cornmeal in a thin stream while whisking continuously.

Reduce the heat to low and simmer, stirring frequently with a whisk, for about 5 minutes or until polenta is smooth and thickened. Remove from the heat and stir in cheese and the remaining 2 tablespoons of butter. Serve immediately or place a piece of plastic wrap directly on top, making contact with the polenta to prevent a film from forming, and just reheat later.

If reheating, add additional stock or water to bring back to a creamy stage. Usually polenta won't remain in the same creamy format if it sits too long, so time accordingly. Serve warm.

Makes approximately 4 to 6 servings

~An umami recipe

My Favorite Pasta Hack

Kids love pasta, but that big pot every day is such a hassle! Parents, this is not a recipe, although I'm sure you will appreciate this dynamic kitchen hack, which will save you time. Cook enough pasta for the whole week at one time!

Here's How

Boil a gallon of water for each pound of pasta in a large pot. Add 1/2 tablespoon salt per gallon. Bring the water to a full boil over high heat. Add the pasta. Stir. Cook the pasta for 5 to 8 minutes or about 2 to 3 minutes less than the package directions. Pasta should be firm to the bite when complete. Do not overcook. Drain water and immediately toss pasta with enough olive oil to lightly coat. This will help keep the pasta's starch from sticking. Portion servings in airtight containers. Use one container for each pasta recipe you have planned midweek. Store in the fridge. Reheat the pasta, add toppings, and dinner is ready.

~Will last up to 4 days airtight.

Chapter Eighteen

ALTERNATIVE DESSERT

In Western culture, dessert is a course consisting of sweet foods that typically comes at the end of a large meal. It was not until the 18th century, when sugar was first manufactured, that people began to enjoy sweets; even then, sugar was so expensive that it was only for the wealthy and for very special occasions.

Today, sugary desserts are often laden with ingredients that should never enter our bodies, and we should only consume sweets on a calorically incremental level. Children, especially picky eaters, should not be bribed with desserts or sweets in order to coax them into eating a balanced meal. Avoiding that habit is half the battle!

Eliminating sugary dessert foods can be a useful strategy to reduce the calories, carbohydrates or fat consumed. Look upon this as an occasion to present healthier options, such as fruits and cheeses. Personally, I avoided serving my family dessert after dinner every evening. We gathered at the table for dessert on occasions relating to celebrations or milestone achievements. Taking dessert off the menu will help your picky eater stay focused on consuming healthier options at mealtimes.

Keep desserts for superfluous times; conversely, if you decide to serve dessert every day, make sure it is healthy and free from processed ingredients. I'd rather children eat organic cane sugar than prepackaged store-bought desserts filled with artificial ingredients, unnatural dyes, and shelf stabilizers.

Homemade Soft-Serve Ice Cream

Chill the kids out fast with this fun, no-hassle activity. Homemade soft serve ice cream is not only fun, it's delicious! Make sure you give each child their own bag filled with the recipe ingredients so there is no fighting!

You'll Need

    1/2 cup milk

    1/2 teaspoon vanilla

    1 tablespoon sugar

    2 tablespoons chocolate sauce (optional)

    4–6 cups ice, crushed

    1/4 cup large rock salt

    2 quart-size ziplock bags

    1 gallon-size ziplock freezer bag

    1 hand towel or pair of gloves

Here's How

Combine the milk, vanilla, sugar and chocolate together in one of the quart bags. Seal tightly. Allow as little air inside as possible. Place this bag inside the other quart bag and seal.

Put the double bagger bag inside the gallon-size bag and fill the big bag with ice. Salt the ice. Remove all the air the best you can. Seal. Wrap the bag in the towel or put gloves on and massage so the ice surrounds the cream mixture and begins to freeze. Depending on your touch, you should have soft serve in 10 to 15 minutes. Add additional freeze time in your freezer for firmer ice cream. Give this tasty task to the kids, and you will actually find time to clean up after mealtime—just make sure the bags are sealed tightly, or you will have more to clean!

Makes 1 serving

Fresh Fruit Galette

This free-form pie-shaped dessert is so easy to make, and kids can get involved too. You can bet you'll use this recipe over and over!

You'll Need

2½ cups all-purpose flour

3 tablespoons sugar

1½ teaspoons table salt

8 ounces butter, frozen, grated

2–3 tablespoons ice cold water

Fruit filling

Filling

4–5 cups fresh berries

1/3 cup sugar

3 tablespoons all-purpose flour

1 tablespoon fresh lemon juice

2 tablespoons butter, cut into cubes

Here's How

In a small bowl or disposable food storage bag, toss the berries with the filling ingredients to coat.

In a large bowl or disposable food storage bag, add all the dough ingredients except the water. Rub the grated butter into the flour until the dough forms pea-size balls and the flour feels and appears close to beach sand. Add the ice water in intervals until the dough comes together similar to Play-Doh. Careful not to overmix.

Remove from the bag onto a clean work surface and press into a wide, flat disc. Return to the bag and seal airtight. Rest in the refrigerator a minimum of 30 minutes. Dust a clean work surface with a little flour, and roll dough to a 12 to 14-inch circle about 1/4-inch thick.

Place the fruit filling in the center, leaving a 2½-inch gap around the edge. Fold the edges toward the center, creating an overlap after each fold. Complete the circle.

Brush with an egg wash. Bake at 425 °F for about 30 minutes or until nicely browned and the fruit mixture is bubbling.

Red Velvet Beet Cupcakes

Looking for a red dessert for Valentine's Day without artificial coloring? Try this easy sugar beet cupcake recipe!

You'll Need

1 cup red sugar beets (freshly cooked, not canned), pureed

1/3 cup coconut oil, slightly heated to pourable state

1 1/4 cup granulated organic sugar

2 teaspoons Madagascar vanilla extract

1¼ cups all-purpose flour

1/4 teaspoon kosher salt

2 tablespoons natural cocoa powder
(not Dutch-processed cocoa)

1½ teaspoons baking powder

1/2 cup almond milk or substitute

Here's How

Preheat the oven to 325 °F. Prepare a muffin tin with cupcake liners and set aside. In a small bowl, sift together the flour, cocoa powder, salt and baking powder. Set aside.

In the bowl of a stand mixer or a large mixing bowl, add the beet puree. Setting the whip attachment to medium-high speed, begin to combine the beet puree with the oil by adding the oil in a slow yet steady stream. Continue until all the oil is incorporated.

Add the sugar and the vanilla extract. Beat an additional minute. Alternate adding the flour mixture and nut milk until completely incorporated into the batter. Continue to beat until combined. Divide among cupcake liners, filling them 3/4 full. Bake for 20 to 25 minutes or until a toothpick comes out clean. Cool and keep in an airtight container. Frost as desired.

Chocolate Avocado Mousse

Chocolate mousse has never been healthier—or faster! When choosing avocados for this chocolate avocado mousse, use the creamy Hass variety.

You'll Need

4 ripe avocados, peeled and pitted

3 tablespoons honey, maple syrup, or optional liquid sweetener (not granulated sugar)

3/4 cup cocoa powder

1/2 teaspoon vanilla extract

Himalayan salt

4–5 tablespoons nut milk

1 cup berries, for garnish (optional)

Cocoa, for dusting

Here's How

Scoop out the meat of the avocados and place into a stand blender or food processor. Add sweetener of choice, cocoa, vanilla, salt and nut milk. Blend until very smooth, about 1 minute. Taste and adjust for sweetness. Add more nut milk if too thick. Place mixture into serving bowls and chill until ready to serve. Top with fresh raspberries and a sprinkle of cocoa.

Makes approximately 4 servings

Additive-Free Homemade Yellow Cake Mix

My easy homemade yellow cake mix doesn't contain shelf stabilizers. Perfection!

You'll Need

1½ cups organic flour

1 cup organic cane sugar

2 teaspoons baking soda

1/4 teaspoon kosher salt

To Bake

3 organic eggs

½ teaspoon organic vanilla extract

1/3 cup healthy oil

1 cup filtered water

Here's How

For cake mix: Combine all cake-mix ingredients. It makes 2½ cups of cake mix, which will yield one 13 x 9 cake. Store it in an airtight container at room temperature for up to 1 month.

To bake: In a medium bowl, combine the cake mix and eggs, vanilla extract, oil and water. Using an electric mixer, beat about 2 minutes on medium speed. Pour batter into a greased and lightly floured cake pan.

Bake in a preheated 350 °F oven for 25 to 30 minutes, or until center springs back to the touch. Cool.

A FINAL WORD

It is my hope you will learn healthy tips and strategies for the future as well as avoid some of the pitfalls that many other parents have encountered. Develop nutritious routines before the battle begins, and dinnertime will be a pleasant experience for everyone.

I realize that each situation is as individual as the child, so you may need to adapt some of the techniques to work for your unique circumstances. Regardless of your approach, consistency is the key to success!

Remember: You're breaking unhealthy habits today and replacing them with behaviors that will ensure a healthy future for your child. Now that you have been introduced to proven strategies for developing healthy eating habits, you can rest assured that your child will get the proper nutrition he needs. Follow through.

Expect some resistance at first, but be firm and continue your path. Your parenting role will become easier if you stick to a repetitive plan of action. Will your child whine or cry and demand her own way? You can count on it!

As new parents, we often worry that we are not actively making the right choices for our children. Toddlers' bodies are precisely calibrated to take in the necessary number of calories they need to grow and thrive. Our job is just to make sure they get the right variety of calories. Stress less and love more. Child raising goes by rapidly; it would be a shame to miss it because you're too busy stressing about every little green pea. Remember, you have one of the most important jobs in the world, so be good to yourself, too!

—Chef Gigi